MW01115408

RECIPE BOOK THAT CURES HANGOVERS

100 RECIPES TO RECOVER YOUR
BODY AND YOUR MIND

JACK BLACK

Disclaimer

The information contained in this eBook is meant to serve as a comprehensive collection of strategies that the author of this eBook has done research about. Summaries, strategies, tips and tricks are only recommendation by the author, and reading this eBook will not guarantee that one's results will exactly mirror the author's results. The author of the eBook has made all reasonable effort to provide current and accurate information for the readers of the eBook. The author and its associates will not be held liable for any unintentional error or omissions that may be found. The material in the eBook may include information by third parties. Third party materials comprise of opinions expressed by their owners. As such, the author of the eBook does not assume responsibility or liability for any third party material or opinions. Whether because of the progression of the internet, or the unforeseen changes in company policy and editorial submission guidelines, what is stated as fact at the time of this writing may become outdated or inapplicable later.

TABLE OF CONTENTS

INTRODUCTION

Hangovers happen. You just pop out for a sophisticated glass of wine with your colleagues. Next thing you know you're on your third, that home-cooked meal turns into a liquid dinner, and when the alarm goes off the next day you wake up cross-eyed and confused.

Whether you're craving a green juice or feel the need to dump your head into a bucket of waffles, these hangover recipes will take you from zero to (nearly a) hero.

The list starts with the good healthy breakfast and progresses to the gooey, greasy, cheesy recipes that will make your hungover soul sing.

BREAKFAST

1. Sunday morning baked eggs

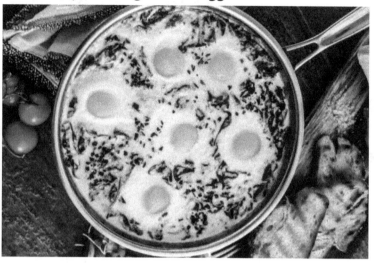

Serves 4

Ingredients

- 4 Tablespoon extra virgin olive oil
- 8 large eggs
- large sprig tarragon, leaves chopped
- 50g gruyere (or vegetarian alternative), grated
- 100ml double cream
- 100g bag watercress, to serve
- Bacon cakes or toast, to serve

Directions

a) Heat oven to 160C/140C fan/gas 3 and bring a kettle of water to the boil.

b) Pour 1 Tablespoon oil into 4 shallow ramekins and crack 2 eggs into each.

c) Season with sea salt and coarse black pepper, sprinkle with the tarragon and cheese, then spoon over the cream.

d) Set the ramekins in a roasting tin, then quarter-fill the tin with water from the kettle.

e) Carefully transfer to the oven and bake for 6-8 minutes.

2. Bacon cakes

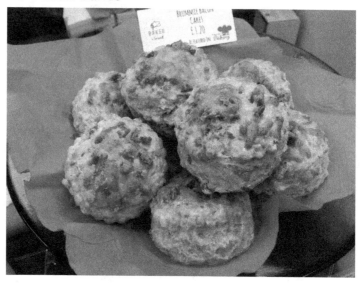

Serves 4

Ingredients

- 3 rashers streaky bacon
- 225g self-rising flour, plus extra for dusting
- 25g butter, cold and cut into small pieces
- 75g mature cheddar, grated
- 150ml milk, plus 2 Tablespoon extra for glazing
- 1 Tablespoon tomato ketchup
- $\frac{1}{2}$ teaspoon Worcestershire sauce

Directions

a) Heat grill to high and grill the bacon for 10 minutes, turning halfway, until crisp.

b) Cool for a few minutes. Meanwhile, heat oven to 180C/160C fan/gas 4 and line a baking sheet with parchment. Sift the flour and $\frac{1}{2}$ teaspoon salt into a bowl, add the butter, then rub in to the texture of fine breadcrumbs. Cut the bacon into small pieces and add to the bowl with a third of the cheese.

c) Mix the milk, ketchup and Worcestershire sauce in a jug. Pour into the bacon mixture, stirring briefly, to make a soft dough. Flour the work surface, turn the dough onto it and shape into an 18cm round. Brush with milk, then cut into 8 wedges with a large knife.

d) Arrange the wedges on the baking sheet and sprinkle with the remaining cheese. Bake for 20-30 minutes or until risen and golden brown, and serve warm.

3. Gorgonzola, bacon & maple toastie

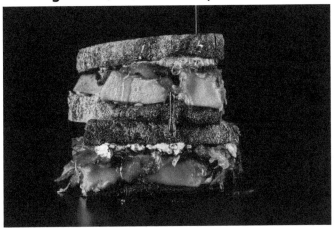

MAKES 4

Ingredients

- 500g pumpkin, peeled, seeds removed, sliced into 4 x 2cm-thick wedges, halved crossways
- 1/3 cup (80ml) light olive oil
- 12 rashers streaky maple-cured bacon (substitute streaky bacon)
- 100g gorgonzola piccante, crumbled
- 200g Monterey Jack cheese, coarsely grated
- 8 x 1cm-thick slices light rye sourdough bread
- 1/4 cup (80g) caramelized onion (from supermarkets)
- 80g unsalted butter, softened
- Maple syrup, to serve

Directions

a) Preheat the oven to 160°C. Grease a baking tray and line with baking paper.
b) Toss pumpkin in a bowl with $\frac{1}{4}$ cup (60ml) oil, 1/2 teaspoon sea salt and a pinch of

black pepper, then place on prepared tray and cover tightly with foil. Roast for 40-50 minutes or until just tender. Remove foil and set aside to cool.

c) Meanwhile, heat remaining 1 Tablespoons oil in a fry-pan over high heat and cook bacon for 3 minutes each side or until golden. Drain on paper towel.

d) To assemble sandwiches, combine cheeses in a bowl. Lay out 4 slices bread and top each evenly with pumpkin. Scatter over caramelised onion, then top with 3 rashers bacon each. Spoon cheese mixture evenly over bacon and top with remaining 4 slices bread.

e) Lightly butter top slices of bread, then flip sandwiches and repeat.

f) Heat a sandwich press and cook the sandwiches for 10 minutes or until golden and cheese has melted. (Rotate sandwiches halfway if using a small press, to ensure they cook evenly.)

g) Using a serrated knife, cut sandwiches in half and drizzle with maple syrup.

4. Beef burgers with provolone & pickles

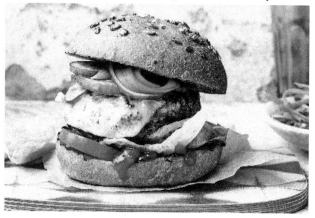

SERVES 4

INGREDIENTS

- 2 slices white bread
- $\frac{1}{2}$ cup (125ml) milk
- 500g beef mince
- 1 egg, lightly beaten
- 2 Tablespoons chopped chives
- $\frac{1}{2}$ cup (40g) finely grated parmesan
- 4 slices provolone cheese
- 4 burger buns, lightly toasted
- Tomato chutney (optional), sliced tomato, and baby cos leaves to serve

Pretty pickles

- $\frac{1}{2}$ cup (125ml) red wine vinegar
- 2 Tablespoons caster sugar
- 1 Tablespoons pink peppercorns, bruised
- $\frac{1}{2}$ Tablespoons fennel seeds, crushed
- $\frac{1}{2}$ bunch each Dutch carrots and radishes, thinly sliced
- 1 small red onion, cut into 5mm rings
- $\frac{1}{2}$ Lebanese cucumber, sliced

Directions

a) For the pretty pickles, place vinegar, sugar, 1/3 cup (80ml) water, peppercorns, fennel seeds and 1 Tablespoons salt flakes into a small saucepan over high heat. Bring to a boil for 1 minute, then cool completely. Place vegetables into a shallow container, pour over liquid to cover and leave 20 minutes.

b) Place bread and milk into a medium bowl. Soak 5 minutes. Gently squeeze bread and discard excess milk. Place bread in a large bowl with mince, egg, chive and parmesan. Season and combine well. Divide mixture into 4 and shape into patties. Place onto a plate, cover and chill 30 minutes to firm up.

c) Heat a barbecue or grill pan over medium-high heat. Cook patties 3 minutes each side or until cooked. Top each with cheese (residual heat will melt it). On each bun base place chutney, tomato, cos, burger, drained pickles and bun lid.

5. Omelet in a Cup

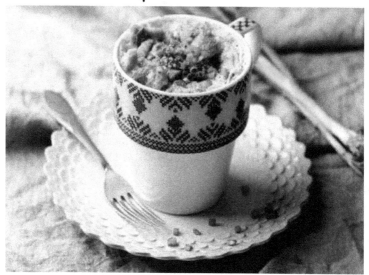

1 serving

Ingredients

- Cooking spray or extra virgin olive oil

- 2 large eggs

- 1 tablespoon milk

- 1 tablespoon grated cheddar cheese

- 1 tablespoon finely chopped red bell pepper

- 1 teaspoon finely chopped chives or green onion

- Pinch salt

- Pinch black pepper

Directions

a) Spray the inside of a large, microwave-safe mug lightly with cooking oil spray.

b) Crack 2 eggs into the mug, add 1 tablespoon of milk, and beat with a fork.

c) Add grated cheese and other extras.

d) Microwave and stir in 20 to 30 second increments:

e) Microwave for 30 second on high. Remove from microwave and stir with a fork.

f) Return to the microwave and cook for another 20 to 30 seconds.

g) You'll see patches of firm cooked egg mixture beginning to form. Remove and stir again.

h) Return to the microwave and cook for another 20 to 30 seconds or until the omelette has set.

6. Grown-up Green Eggs and Ham

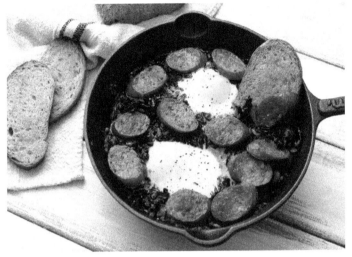

Ingredients

- 1 cup fresh basil leaves
- 2 tablespoons pistachios, chopped
- 1 garlic clove, minced
- $\frac{1}{4}$ cup plus 2 tablespoons extra-virgin olive oil, divided
- $\frac{1}{4}$ cup grated Parmesan cheese
- $\frac{1}{2}$ cup chopped thick-cut ham steak
- 2 large eggs
- 1 to 2 tablespoons chopped flat leaf parsley

Directions

a) Make the Pesto. Combine the first three ingredients in a food processor and pulse until finely chopped. With the food processor running, slowly stream in oil until pesto comes together (you may not need to use exactly $\frac{1}{2}$ cup). Pulse in the grated parmesan cheese until just combined. Reserve three tablespoons pesto and refrigerate the remaining amount in an air-tight container for a week.

b) Brown the ham. In a large nonstick skillet, heat 1 tablespoon oil over medium-high heat. Add chopped ham and sauté until golden brown. Remove from pan and reserve.

c) Scramble the eggs. Heat remaining 1 tablespoon of oil in the same skillet over medium heat. Meanwhile, whisk together eggs and 3 tablespoons reserved pesto in a small bowl. Pour eggs into the pan and shake the pan while stirring the eggs. Cook for 1 minute, stir in reserved ham. Continue cooking for 2 minutes longer, if you're not a fan of soft scrambled eggs.

d) Put it all together. Remove the pan from the heat and stir in flat leaf parsley. Pile the eggs on a crispy piece of toast and eat up.

7. Swedish hash meal

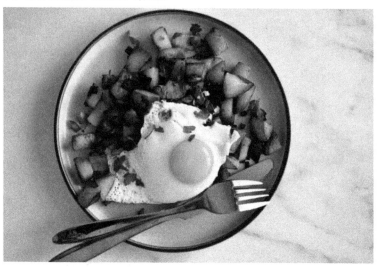

Servings: 5

Ingredients

- 1 & 1/2 Tablespoon olive oil
- 1/2 kg potatoes, peeled and diced
- 1 medium onion, sliced finely
- 5 ounces smoked pork, diced
- 5 ounces ham, diced (about 1/2 cup, heaping)
- 10 ounces sausage, diced (about 300 grams)
- salt and pepper, for seasoning
- parsley, chopped roughly for garnish

Directions

a) Place a medium or large skillet over medium-high heat, then add oil.
b) Once the oil is hot, add the diced potatoes.
c) Cook until the potatoes are halfway done.
d) Add the onions, salt, and pepper.
e) Adjust the heat to medium and cook for about 4 minutes or until the onions have softened.
f) Add the smoked pork, ham, and sausage.
g) Cook until the potatoes are ready, simultaneously checking and adjusting the seasoning during this time.
h) Take the pan off the heat and transfer into plates.
i) Serve with some pickled beets and fried egg.

8. Avocado and Egg Toast

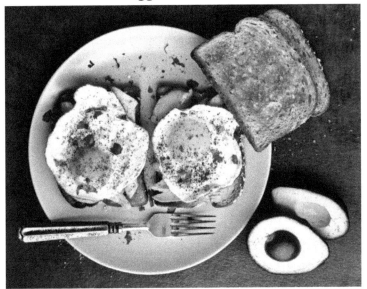

Ingredients

- $\frac{1}{4}$ avocado seeded and peeled
- 1 slice whole grain bread or bread of choice
- Sea salt to taste
- Freshly cracked black pepper to taste
- Fried Eggs
- $\frac{1}{2}$ tablespoon butter
- 1 egg
- Scrambled Eggs
- $\frac{1}{2}$ tablespoon butter
- 2 eggs
- Boiled Eggs
- 2 eggs
- Poached Eggs
- 2 teaspoons white vinegar
- 1 egg

Directions

a) Toast the bread in a toaster until golden and crispy, place the quarter avocado over the toast, slice it and mash it on top of the toast. Top with eggs of choice, and season with salt and pepper, to taste.

b) For fried eggs: Heat butter in nonstick skillet over medium-high heat until hot. Break the egg onto the skillet and immediately reduce the heat to low. Cook uncovered until whites are completely set and yolks are thickened to your liking, about 5-7 minutes.

c) For scrambled eggs: Heat butter in nonstick skillet over medium-high heat until hot. Whisk the eggs in small bowl, then carefully pour into the center of the pan. When the edges start to set, start to gently fold the eggs until the eggs are cooked through, about 2-3 minutes.

d) For boiled eggs: Place the eggs in a saucepan. Pour cool water over the eggs until fully submerged. Bring the water to a rolling boil, then reduce the heat to low and cook according to the desired doneness: 4 minutes for SOFT boiled; 6 minutes for MEDIUM boiled; 12 minutes for HARD boiled. Prepare a bowl of ice water. Transfer the cooked eggs to the ice water to cool completely before peeling.

e) For poached eggs: Bring a large pot of water to a boil. Crack one egg into a small bowl. Stir vinegar into the water and create a vortex with the boiling water. Lower the heat so the water creates a rolling boil at the bottom of the pot. Then, carefully add the egg to the middle of the pot and cook for 3-4 minutes, according to desired doneness. Remove the egg with a slotted spoon.

9. Bacon, Egg, and Cheese Muffin

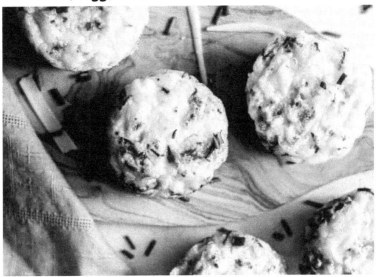

Ingredients

- 5 large eggs
- 1/4 lb. (125g) crisp-cooked bacon, crumbled
- 1 cup grated cheddar, or any cheese you like
- Salt and fresh cracked pepper, to taste
- 1/2 teaspoon Italian seasoning
- 1/2 teaspoon crushed chili pepper flakes

Directions

a) To make the cheesy bacon egg muffins: Preheat your oven to 400°F (200°C).

b) Grease a 6 count muffin pan with oil or non-stick cooking spray. Set aside. In a large mixing bowl, crack in eggs and whisk together with salt and black pepper.

c) Stir in cooked bacon, cheddar cheese, Italian seasoning, and red chili pepper flakes (if using).

d) Divide evenly into muffin cups filling each about 2/3 full. Top with more bacon and cheese if you like. Bake the egg muffins in preheated oven for 12-15 minutes, or until set.

10. Bacon and Egg Breakfast Casserole

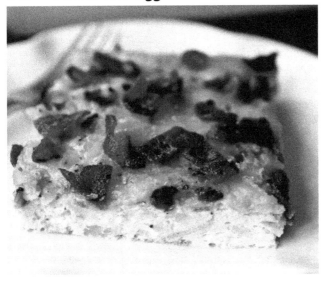

SERVINGS 10

Ingredients

- 1 lb. bacon, cut into 1/2-inch strips
- 1 yellow onion diced
- 1 red bell pepper seeds removed and diced
- 3 cloves garlic minced
- 12 large eggs
- 1 cup milk
- 3 cups frozen diced potatoes you don't have to thaw or cook the potatoes
- 2 cups shredded cheddar cheese divided
- 1 1/2 teaspoons salt
- 1/2 teaspoon black pepper
- 2 green onions chopped

Directions

a) Heat the oven to 350°F. Grease a 9x13 baking dish with nonstick cooking spray and set aside.

b) In a large skillet, cook bacon over medium heat, stirring occasionally. Cook until it is a nice crispy brown. Remove bacon with a slotted spoon and place on a paper towel lined plate. Roughly chop the bacon and set aside.

c) Add the onion and red pepper to the skillet and cook over medium heat until tender. Add the garlic and cook for 2 minutes. Set aside.

d) In a large bowl, beat the eggs and whisk in the milk. Stir in the cooked vegetables, potatoes, and 1 cup of the shredded cheese. Set $\frac{3}{4}$ cup of bacon aside and stir in the rest. Season with salt and pepper.

e) Pour the mixture into the prepared baking dish and top remaining cheese and green onions. Bake for 20 minutes so the eggs start to set up. Carefully add the remaining bacon to the top of the casserole. Bake for an additional 20 to 30 minutes or until the eggs are firm and the top is slightly golden brown. Let stand for 10 minutes. Cut into squares and serve warm.

11. Caribbean Oats Porridge

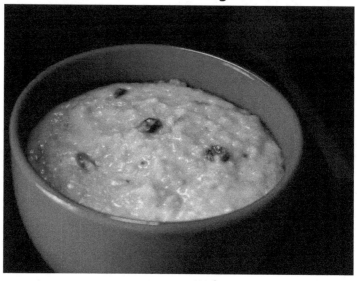

Ingredients
- 1 cup rolled oats
- 3 cups water, divided
- 1 stick cinnamon stick
- 1/4 cup raisins, rinsed
- 1/2 teaspoon freshly grated nutmeg
- 2 tablespoons sugar, more to taste
- 1/4 cup whole milk, more to taste

Directions
a) Soak the oats in 1 cup of water for 4 minutes.
b) While the oats are soaking, bring the remaining 2 cups of water and the cinnamon stick to a boil in medium heat.
c) When the water boils, add the soaked oats along with any residual soaking liquid.
d) Stir in the rinsed raisins and reduce to low heat.
e) Cover the pot and cook for 5 to 6 minutes or until the mixture becomes very thick.
f) Remove from the heat and discard the cinnamon stick. Stir in the freshly grated nutmeg, sugar, and whole milk.

12.   Blueberry Vanilla Quinoa Bowl

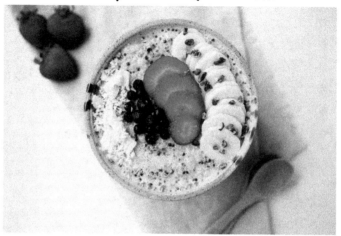

Yield 4

Ingredients
- 1 cup quinoa
- 2 cups water
- 1 tablespoon vanilla
- 2 cups blueberries fresh or frozen
- 1 tablespoon coconut oil melted
- 1/2 teaspoon cinnamon
- sea salt to taste

Directions
a) Preheat oven to 400 degrees F.
b) Combine the quinoa, water, and vanilla in a saucepan with a pinch of salt. Bring to a boil, cover, and reduce heat to low. Simmer for 15 minutes until liquid is absorbed.
c) Toss the blueberries with the coconut oil and cinnamon. Spread on a parchment-lined baking sheet (don't skip the parchment!) Roast until soft and bubbly, about 15 minutes.
d) Serve the quinoa topped with the roasted blueberries. Top with a few fresh blueberries, coconut, or slivered almonds if desired.

13. Maple Cinnamon Breakfast Quinoa

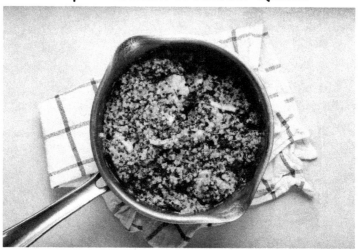

Ingredients

- 1 cup quinoa
- 2 to 2 1/2 cups water
- 2/3 cup soy milk
- 1 teaspoon vegan margarine
- 1/2 teaspoon ground cinnamon
- 2 tablespoons maple syrup
- 2 tablespoons raisins, optional
- 2 medium bananas, sliced, optional

Directions

a) Heat the quinoa and water in a small saucepan and bring to a boil. Reduce to a simmer and allow to cook, covered, for 15 minutes, until liquid is absorbed.

b) Remove from heat and fluff the quinoa with a fork. Cover, and allow to sit for 5 minutes.

c) Stir in the margarine and soy milk, then remaining ingredients.

d) Serve and enjoy.

14.   Apple Bacon Muffins

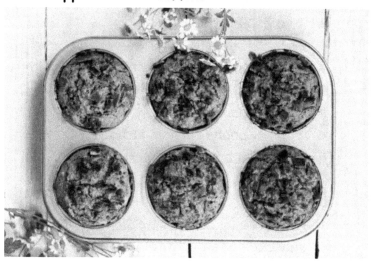

Servings:
12 to 15 servings

Ingredients

- 4 ounces (1/2 cup) butter (softened)
- 1/2 cup packed brown sugar
- 2 large eggs
- 2 teaspoons baking powder
- 1/2 teaspoon salt
- 2 cups all-purpose flour
- 2 tablespoons cinnamon
- 2/3 cup milk
- 3/4 cup finely chopped apple
- 1/2 cup diced cooked and drained bacon

Directions

a) Heat the oven to 375 F.

b) Spray muffin cups with nonstick baking spray or cooking spray.

c) In a large mixing bowl with an electric mixer, cream butter and brown sugar until light. Beat in the eggs until well blended.

d) In a separate bowl, combine the flour, baking powder, salt, and cinnamon; stir or whisk to blend thoroughly.

e) Add the dry ingredients to the creamed mixture, alternating with the milk. Stir just until blended. Fold in the apple and bacon until blended.

f) Immediately spoon the batter into the prepared muffin pan, filling the cups about three-quarters full.

g) Bake for 18 to 22 minutes, until lightly browned.

h) Cool in the pan for about 10 minutes, then remove to a rack to cool completely.

15.　Raisin Bran Muffins

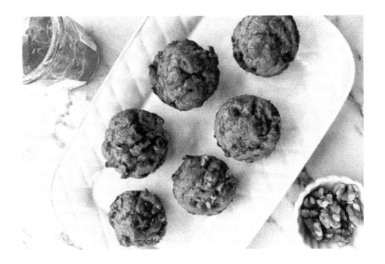

Makes 6

Ingredients
- 1/4 cup vegetable oil, plus more for tin
- 1 1/2 cups raisin bran cereal
- 3/4 cup milk
- 1/2 cup whole-wheat flour
- 1/2 cup all-purpose flour
- 2 teaspoons baking powder
- 1/2 teaspoon ground cinnamon
- 1/4 teaspoon salt
- 1 large egg, lightly beaten
- 1/4 cup packed dark-brown sugar

Directions

a) Preheat oven to 400. Lightly oil a 6-cup standard muffin tin, or use paper liners. In a medium bowl, combine cereal and milk; let stand until softened, about 5 minutes. In a small bowl, whisk together flours, baking powder, cinnamon, and salt.

b) Stir oil, egg, and sugar into cereal mixture. Fold in flour mixture. Divide batter among cups. Bake until a toothpick inserted in the center of a muffin comes out clean, 20 to 25 minutes.

c) Cool in tin 5 minutes, then turn out onto a wire rack; let cool completely, or serve warm.

d) Store up to 5 days at room temperature in a resealable plastic bag.

16. Strawberry spinach salad

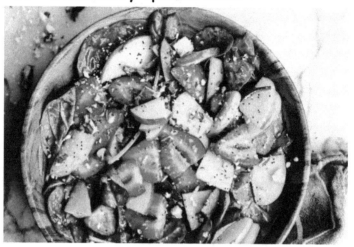

Servings: 4

Ingredients

- 2 tablespoons sesame seeds
- 1 tablespoon poppy seeds
- $\frac{1}{2}$ cup white sugar
- $\frac{1}{2}$ cup olive oil
- $\frac{1}{4}$ cup distilled white vinegar
- $\frac{1}{4}$ teaspoon paprika
- $\frac{1}{4}$ teaspoon Worcestershire sauce
- 1 tablespoon minced onion
- 10 ounces fresh spinach - rinsed, dried and torn into bite-size pieces
- 1 quart strawberries - cleaned, hulled and sliced
- $\frac{1}{4}$ cup almonds, blanched and slivered

Directions

a) In a medium bowl, whisk together the sesame seeds, poppy seeds, sugar, olive oil, vinegar, paprika, Worcestershire sauce and onion. Cover, and chill for one hour.

b) In a large bowl, combine the spinach, strawberries and almonds. Pour dressing over salad, and toss. Refrigerate 10 to 15 minutes before serving.

17.   Polish Zapiekanka

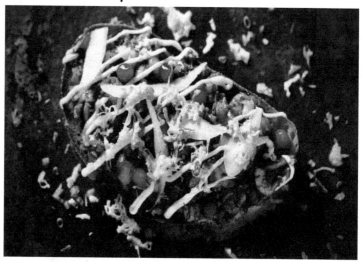

yield: 2

Ingredients
- 1 baguette
- 10 oz. (300g) button mushrooms
- 1 small onion
- 5 oz. (150g) mild cheese (e.g. gouda)
- 1 Tablespoon canola oil (for frying)
- 2 Tablespoon tomato ketchup

Directions
a) Preheat the oven to 400°F (200°C).
b) Cut the baguette lengthwise. Scoop it out a bit.
c) Wash the mushrooms, dry them and chop into small pieces.
d) Peel the onion and chop into small pieces.
e) Add oil to the frying pan. Sauté the chopped onion and mushrooms for 7-10 minutes. Season with salt and pepper.
f) Grate the cheese.
g) Fill the baguettes with fried onion and mushrooms. Cover with grated cheese.
h) Bake until golden (approx.8-10 minutes).
i) Serve with ketchup.

18. Tofu & Kales scramble

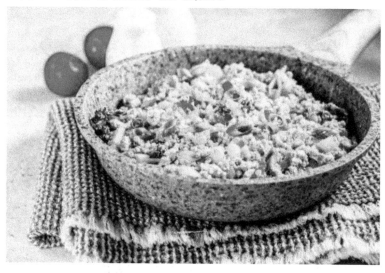

Servings 2

Ingredients

- 8 ounces extra-firm tofu
- 1-2 Tablespoon olive oil
- 1/4 red onion (thinly sliced)
- 1/2 red pepper (thinly sliced)
- 2 cups kale (loosely chopped)

Sauce

- 1/2 Tablespoon sea salt (reduce amount for less salty sauce)
- 1/2 Tablespoon garlic powder
- 1/2 Tablespoon ground cumin
- 1/4 Tablespoon chili powder
- Water (to thin)
- 1/4 Tablespoon turmeric (optional)

For serving (optional)

- Salsa
- Cilantro
- Hot Sauce

Directions

a) Pat tofu dry and roll in a clean, absorbent towel with something heavy on top, such as a cast-iron skillet, for 15 minutes.

b) While tofu is draining, prepare sauce by adding dry spices to a small bowl and adding enough water to make a pourable sauce. Set aside.

c) Prep veggies and warm a large skillet over medium heat. Once hot, add olive oil and the onion and red pepper. Season with a pinch each salt and pepper and stir. Cook until softened – about 5 minutes.

d) Add kale, season with a bit more salt and pepper, and cover to steam for 2 minutes.

e) In the meantime, unwrap tofu and use a fork to crumble into bite-sized pieces.

f) Use a spatula to move the veggies to one side of the pan and add tofu. Sauté for 2 minutes, then add sauce, pouring it mostly over the tofu and a little over the veggies.

g) Stir immediately, evenly distributing the sauce. Cook for another 5-7 minutes until tofu is slightly browned.

19. Apple cereal

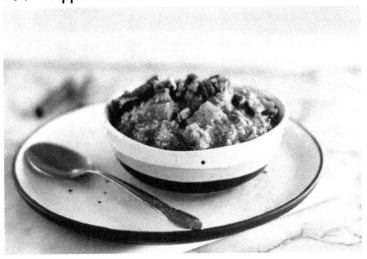

1 serving

Ingredients:

- 1 apple
- 1 pear
- 2 sticks celery
- 1 tablespoon water
- optional: cinnamon

Directions

a) Cut the apple, pear, and celery into pieces and put in a blender.
b) Blend fruit and vegetables with water to a smooth consistency.
c) Spice it up with cinnamon if you like.

APPETIZERS & SNACKS

20. Okra & Cucumber Bites

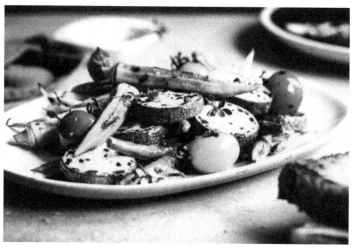

Serves 4

Ingredients
- 11/2 pounds okra, rinsed and dried
- 1 large cucumber
- 1 teaspoon red chili powder
- 1/2 teaspoon Warm Spice Mix
- teaspoon dry mango powder
- 31/2 tablespoons chickpea flour
- cups vegetable oil
- 1 teaspoon Chaat Spice Mix
- Table salt, to taste

Directions

a) Remove the stems from the okra. Cut each piece lengthwise into 4 pieces. Lay out the pieces in large, flat dish; set aside. Slice the cucumber

b) In a small mixing bowl, mix together the red chili powder, spice mix, and dry mango powder. Sprinkle this mixture over the okra. Toss well to ensure that all the pieces are covered with the spice powder. Sprinkle the chickpea flour over the okra. Toss again to ensure that each piece is lightly and evenly covered.

c) In a deep pan, add the vegetable oil to about 1 inch deep. Heat the oil over high heat until smoking, about 370°. Reduce the heat to medium-high.

d) Add some of the okra and deep-fry until well browned, about 4 minutes. Remove with a slotted spoon and place on a paper towel to drain. Continue until all of the okra is fried. Let the oil return to its smoking point between batches.

e) Sprinkle the spice mix on the okra and cucumber. Toss well and season with salt. Serve immediately.

21. Fenugreek-Flavored Meatballs

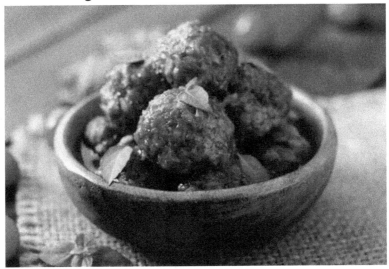

Serves 4

Ingredients

- 1/2-pound ground lean lamb
- 1 small onion, minced
- tablespoon dried fenugreek leaves
- 1/4 teaspoon Ginger-Garlic Paste
- teaspoons Warm Spice Mix
- teaspoons fresh lemon juice
- Table salt, to taste
- 2 tablespoons vegetable oil
- Red onion rings, for garnish

Directions

a) Preheat oven to 500°, or turn on the broiler.

b) In a mixing bowl, combine all of the ingredients except the oil and red onion rings. Mix well, using your hands.

c) Divide the mixture into 8 equal parts and roll into balls. Using a pastry brush, brush the meatballs with the oil. Place all the meatballs on a baking sheet in a single layer.

d) Place the baking sheet under a hot broiler or in the oven and cook for 8 to 10 minutes, turning frequently until the meatballs are well browned on all sides and the meat is completely cooked through.

e) Garnish with red onion rings and serve hot.

22.Sweet potatoes with Tamarind

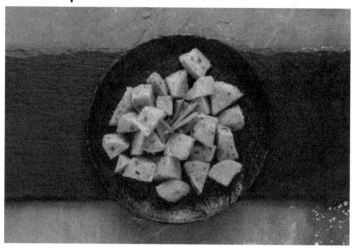

Serves 4

Ingredients

- 4 small sweet potatoes
- 11/2 tablespoons Tamarind
- Chutney
- 1/4 teaspoon black salt
- 1 tablespoon fresh lemon juice
- 1/2 teaspoon cumin seeds, roasted and roughly pounded

Directions

a) Peel the sweet potatoes and cut them into 1/2-inch cubes. Cook in salted water to cover for 5 to 8 minutes or until just fork-tender. Drain and let cool.

b) Put all the ingredients in a bowl and toss gently. Scoop the sweet sweet potatoes in equal portions into 4 bowls. Stick a few toothpicks into the cubed sweet sweet potatoes and serve.

22. Ginger Chicken Bites

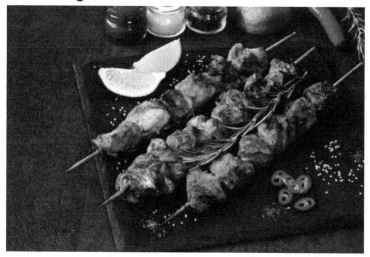

Serves 4

Ingredients
- 1 tablespoons grated ginger-root
- 1 teaspoon fresh lemon juice
- tablespoon vegetable oil
- 1/2 teaspoon red chili powder
- Table salt, to taste
- 11/2 pounds boneless chicken breast
- 2 tablespoons vegetable oil
- Lemon wedges, for garnish

Directions
a) In a bowl or resealable plastic bag, combine the grated ginger, lemon juice, oil, red chili powder, and salt; mix well.
b) Add the chicken cubes. Marinate, covered and refrigerated, for 5 to 6 hours or, preferably, overnight.
c) Preheat oven to 425°.
d) Thread the chicken onto skewers and baste with the vegetable oil. Place the chicken on a foil-lined baking sheet and bake for about 7 minutes.
e) Turn once and baste with any remaining oil. Bake for another 7 minutes.
f) Serve hot, garnished with lemon wedges.

23.   Almond bars

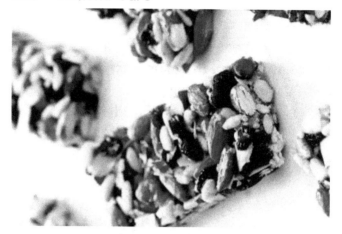

4 bars

Ingredients:

- 1 ½ cup almonds
- ½ cup shredded coconut
- 1 teaspoon cinnamon
- 1 pinch cardamom
- 1 pinch ginger
- 3 dates
- 5 apricots, soaked

Directions

a) Pulse the almonds to a fine flour in a small food processor.
b) Add the coconut and spices and continue blending. Add dates and apricots and continue until all is blended.
c) Shape into rectangular bars—this will be easier with the help of parchment paper!

24. Apple sandwich with goji berries

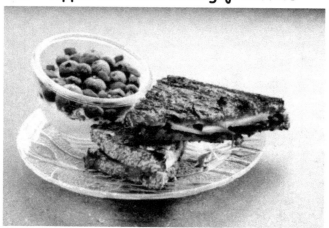

2 servings

Ingredients:

- $\frac{1}{2}$ cup (100 ml) sesame seeds
- 1-2 tablespoons your choice of oil
- 1 tablespoon desiccated coconut1 tablespoon coconut oil
- 2 tablespoons goji berries

Directions

a) Soften the coconut oil.
b) Mix the sesame seeds in the blender until they are finely ground, add 1 to 2 tablespoons oil, and blend again until you have a smooth paste.
c) Mix the sesame paste with coconut flakes and coconut oil.
d) Cut the apples into slices and spread them with tahini. Top with goji berries.

25. Fig Stuffed Pears

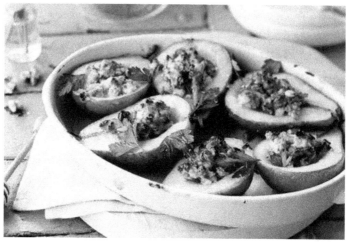

2 servings

Ingredients:

- $\frac{1}{4}$ cup (50 ml) walnuts
- 5 figs, soaked
- $\frac{1}{2}$ teaspoon cinnamon
- $\frac{1}{2}$-$\frac{3}{4}$inch (1-2 cm) of fresh ginger, grated
- 2 teaspoons lemon juice
- 1 pinch nutmeg
- $\frac{1}{4}$-$\frac{1}{2}$cup (50-100 ml) soaking water from figs
- 1 pear

Directions

a) Pulse the walnuts in a food processor.
b) Add the figs and continue blending. Add the remaining ingredients and mix until well blended.
c) Cut the pear into slices and spread the mixture on them.

26. Blackberries with Brazil nut

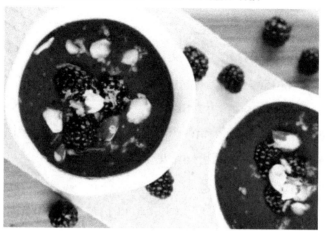

1 serving

Ingredients:

- $\frac{1}{2}$ cup (100 ml) Brazil nuts
- $1\frac{1}{2}$ cups (300 ml) water
- $\frac{1}{4}$ cup (50 ml) blackberries, frozen or semi-thawed
- 1 tablespoon acai powder (optional)
- 2 apricots, soaked1 pinch salt

Directions

a) Mix Brazil nuts in water to a milky consistency and strain through wire strainer.

b) Blend with all other ingredients until you have a smoothie.

27. Spice balls

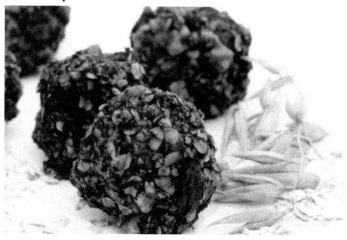

10-15 balls

Ingredients:

- 1 scant cup (200 ml) almonds
- 1½ cups (300 ml) sunflower seeds
- ½ cup (100 ml) pumpkin seeds
- 2 teaspoons ground ginger
- 2 teaspoons ground cloves
- 2 tablespoons cinnamon
- a pinch of salt
- ¼ cup (50 ml) coconut oil
- 1¾ cup (400 ml) raisins, soaked

Directions

a) Pulse almonds, sunflower seeds, and pumpkin seeds in food processor until they are finely minced. Add spices and salt and process again.

b) Add the coconut and raisins, and process until well blended. Squeeze into balls and refrigerate. The coconut oil will make the balls solidify.

28. Celery snack

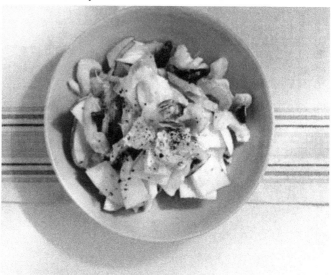

1 serving

Ingredients:

- 1 apple
- celery stalk
- $\frac{1}{4}$ cup (50 ml) walnuts, soaked

Directions

a) Cut the apple and celery into small pieces and roughly chop the walnuts.

b) Mix all ingredients together.

29. Spirulina balls

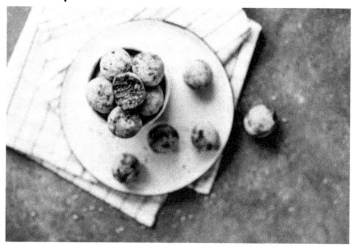

10-15 balls

Ingredients:

- 3 cups (700 ml) hazelnuts
- 1½ cups (300 ml) raisins, soaked
- 2 tablespoons coconut oil, grated lemon zest from 2 lemons
- 1 tablespoon spirulina powder

Directions

a) Pulse the hazelnuts in a food processor until they are ground. Add the raisins and process again.
b) Add the coconut oil, lemon zest, and spirulina powder. Roll into bite-sized balls, or eat as is.

SOUPS

30. Czech Garlic Soup

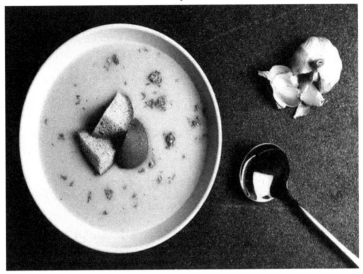

Servings: 4

Ingredients

- $\frac{1}{2}$ tablespoon unsalted butter
- 6 to 8 cloves garlic, crushed (you can use even more, if you'd like!)
- 6 cups chicken, beef, or vegetable broth or stock
- Kosher salt and freshly ground black pepper
- 1 pound (about 2 medium to large) waxy potatoes (white, yellow, or red-not russets), peeled and diced
- 1 teaspoon dried marjoram
- 1 teaspoon caraway seeds
- 1 large egg, beaten (optional)
- 3 ounces (3 to 4 slices) rye bread, cubed
- 1 teaspoon olive oil or olive oil spray
- 4 ounces cubed cheese, Emmental, Gruyere, or Camembert-rind removed (optional)
- 2 tablespoons finely chopped parsley

Directions

a) Melt the butter in a medium pan over medium heat, and add the garlic.

b) Cook until softened and aromatic, about 4 to 5 minutes. Add the broth and bring to a boil over high heat.

c) When boiling, season with salt and pepper, then add the diced potatoes, marjoram, and caraway seeds. Reduce heat and simmer, covered for 15 to 20 minutes until the potatoes are tender. Adjust seasoning as needed.

d) If you are adding an egg, pour it in slowly while mixing the soup to create ribbons of cooked egg.

e) Meanwhile, heat an oven or toaster oven to 350°F. Add the cubed rye bread to a small sheet pan and either drizzle with olive oil or spray with olive oil spray, and toss with your hands to coat.

f) Toast for about 10 to 15 minutes, stirring occasionally, until golden brown and crispy.

g) Serve the soup topped with croutons and parsley, and if desired stir in some cheese.

31.   Hangover soup

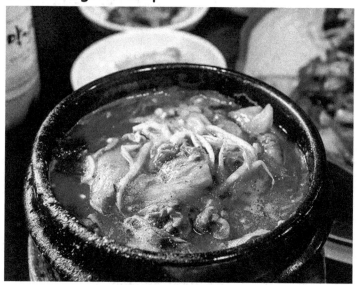

Yield: 6 servings

Ingredient

- ½ pounds Polish sausage; thinly slice
- 2 Slices bacon
- 1 Onion; chopped
- 1 Green pepper; chopped
- 4 cups Beef broth
- 1 can 16-ounce sauerkraut; rinsed;
- 1 cup Sliced fresh mushrooms
- 2 Stalks celery; sliced
- 2 Tomatoes; chopped
- 2 teaspoons Paprika
- 1 teaspoon Caraway seed
- ½ cup Sour cream
- 2 tablespoons Flour

Directions

a) In Dutch oven; cook sausage and bacon until sausage is brown and bacon is crisp. Remove sausage and bacon, and drain; reserve drippings. Crumble bacon. To drippings add onion and green pepper; cook until tender but not brown. Drain off fat. Stir in cooked sausage and bacon, beef broth, sauerkraut, mushrooms, celery, tomatoes, paprika and caraway seed. Bring to boiling; reduce heat.

b) Cover and simmer 45 minutes. Meanwhile, combine sour cream and flour.

c) Gradually stir about 1 cup of the hot soup into sour cream mixture.

d) Return all to Dutch oven. Cook and stir until thickened and bubbly.

e) Cook and stir 1 minute more.

32. Korean Hangover Soup

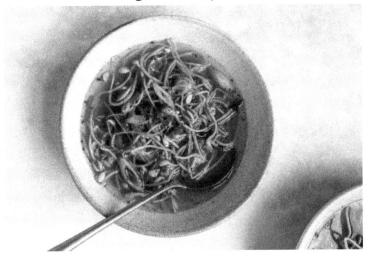

Ingredients

- 1 kg of beef bone
- Water

Directions

a) Soak the beef bones cold water for at least 1 hour to draw out the blood. Rinse the bones in cold water.

b) Place the bones in a large pot filled with boiling water. Boil for 5-10 minutes. Then drain out this water, to get rid of the excess fat and impurities.

c) Add clean water again to the bones. Simmer for at least for a day, until you get a milky and thick broth.

d) Chill the broth for several hours. You can see fat floats to the top and gets hardened. Remove the solid fat from the top.

33. Beetroot Soup

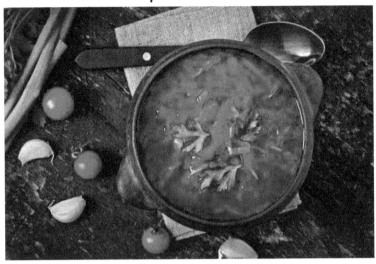

Ingredients

- 1 large beetroot
- 1 cup water
- 2 pinch cumin powder
- 2 pinch pepper
- 1 pinch cinnamon
- 4 pinch salt
- Squeeze of lemon
- $\frac{1}{2}$ Tablespoon ghee

Directions

a) Boil the beetroot then peel.

b) Blend with the water and filter if desired.

c) Boil the mixture then add the remaining ingredients and serve.

34.   Mixed Dal Soup

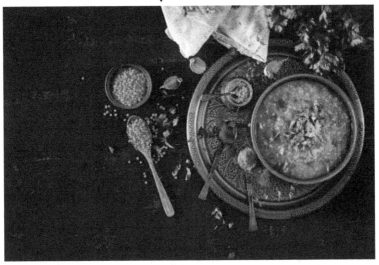

Ingredients

- 1/2 cup dal
- 1 $\frac{1}{2}$ cups water
- $\frac{1}{2}$ Tablespoon turmeric
- 1 Tablespoon oil
- $\frac{1}{2}$ Tablespoon mustard seeds
- $\frac{1}{2}$ Tablespoon cumin seeds
- 5-6 curry leaves
- $\frac{1}{2}$ Tablespoon ginger – grated
- $\frac{1}{2}$ Tablespoon coriander powder
- Pinch asafetida
- Fresh grated coconut - optional
- Salt and jaggery/brown sugar to taste
- Fresh coriander

Directions

a) Place water and dal in a large pot or pressure cooker and add turmeric. Bring to the boil and cook until the dal is soft.

a) In a separate pan heat, the oil, add the mustard seeds, then cumin seeds, curry leaves, ginger, coriander powder and asafoetida.

b) Add coconut, salt and jaggery to taste.

c) Garnish with fresh coriander and coconut.

35.   Dome-Soothing Soup

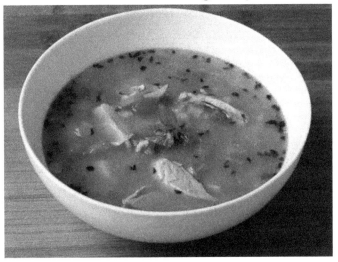

Ingredients

- 1 tablespoon extra-virgin olive oil
- 1 yellow onion, diced
- 2 cloves garlic, minced
- 2 (9-ounce) bags baby spinach
- 1 handful fresh mint, roughly chopped
- 2 slices ginger, about the size of a quarter, peeled (optional)
- 1 cup chicken stock (use vegetable stock or water to make this vegetarian)
- 2 pinches salt

Directions

a) Heat the oil in a pot over medium heat. Add onion and garlic and cook until onion is translucent. Be careful not to burn the garlic. Add spinach, mint, and ginger, if using.

b) As the spinach starts to wilt, add stock or water and salt. When the spinach is completely cooked, remove from heat.

c) Blend with an immersion blender, or put in a blender in batches, and puree until smooth.

36.   White Pumpkin & Coconut Soup

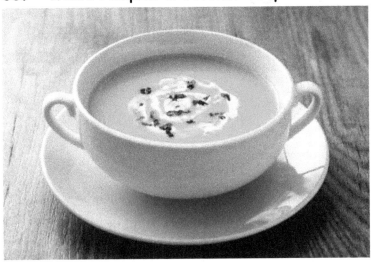

Ingredients
- 1 medium size white pumpkin
- cumin seeds
- curry leaves
- Fresh coriander leaves
- Salt and sugar to taste
- Coconut to taste

Directions
a) Boil the gourd then blend to a liquid.
b) Mix the gourd pulp and water (saved from boiling) to the thickness desired.
c) Add cumin seeds and curry leaves.
d) Add sugar and salt to taste. Bring to the boil.
e) Garnish with fresh coriander leaves and coconut.

37. Whole Mung Soup

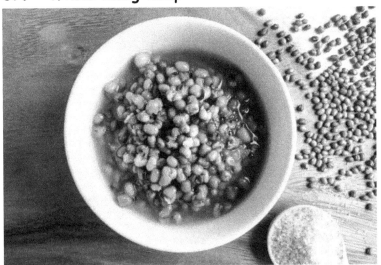

Ingredients
- ½ cup mung beans, whole
- 1 cup water
- ¼ Tablespoon cumin powder
- 4-6 drops of lemon
- ½ Tablespoon vegetable oil/ghee - optional
- Salt to taste

Directions
a) Soak the mung beans overnight or for 10 hours.
b) Boil the mung beans in the water or in a pressure cooker (2 whistles) till soft.
c) Blend mung beans and water together until smooth. Bring to the boil.
d) Add lemon, cumin powder, ghee and salt.

38. Golden Turmeric Cauliflower Soup

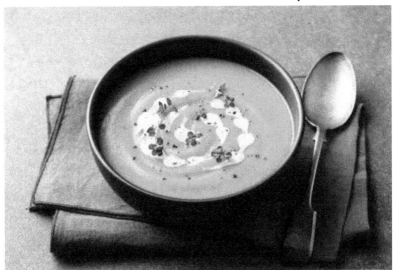

Ingredients

- 6 heaping cups cauliflower florets
- 3 garlic cloves, minced
- 2 Tablespoon plus 1 Tablespoon grape seed, coconut, or avocado oil, divided
- 1 Tablespoon turmeric
- 1 Tablespoon ground cumin
- $\frac{1}{8}$ Tablespoon crushed red pepper flakes
- 1 medium yellow onion or fennel bulb, chopped
- 3 cups vegetable broth
- $\frac{1}{4}$ cup full-fat coconut milk, shaken, to serve

Directions

a) Heat the oven to 450°. In a large bowl, toss cauliflower and garlic with 2 Tablespoon oil, until well coated.

b) Add turmeric, cumin, and red pepper flakes, and toss to coat evenly. Spread cauliflower on a baking sheet in a single layer, and bake until browned and tender, 25-30 minutes.

c) Meanwhile, in a large pot or Dutch oven, heat remaining 1 Tablespoon oil over medium heat. Add onion, and cook for 2-3 minutes, until translucent.

d) When cauliflower is done baking, remove from the oven. Reserve 1 cup to top soup. Take remaining cauliflower and add to a medium pot with onion, and pour in vegetable broth. Bring to a boil, then cover and cook over low heat, 15 minutes.

e) Blend soup to a smooth purée using an immersion blender, or let it cool and purée in batches with a regular blender.

f) Serve topped with reserved roasted cauliflower and a drizzle of coconut milk.

39. Immunity Soup

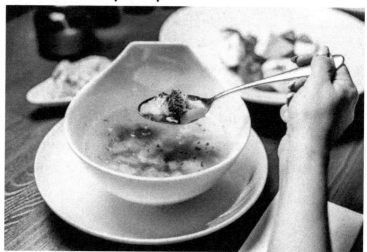

Yield Serves 8

Ingredients

- 2 tablespoons olive oil
- 1 1/2 cups chopped onion
- 3 celery stalks, thinly sliced
- 2 large carrots, thinly sliced
- 1-pound pre-sliced vitamin D-enhanced mushrooms
- 10 medium garlic cloves, minced
- 8 cups unsalted chicken stock
- 4 thyme sprigs
- 2 bay leaves 1 (15-oz.) can unsalted chickpeas, drained
- 2 pounds skinless, bone-in chicken breasts
- 1 1/2 teaspoons kosher salt
- 1/2 teaspoon crushed red pepper
- 12 ounces curly kale, stems removed, leaves torn

Directions

a) Heat oil in a large Dutch oven over medium heat

b) Add onion, celery, and carrots; cook, stirring occasionally, 5 minutes. Add mushrooms and garlic; cook, stirring often, 3 minutes. Stir in stock, thyme, bay leaves, and chickpeas; bring to a simmer. Add chicken, salt, and red pepper; cover and simmer until chicken is done, about 25 minutes.

c) Remove chicken from Dutch oven; cool slightly. Shred meat with 2 forks; discard bones. Stir chicken and kale into soup; cover and simmer until kale is just tender, about 5 minutes. Discard thyme sprigs and bay leaves.

40. Spinach soup

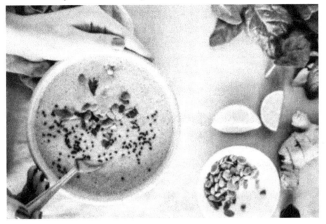

Serves 2

- 4 inches (10 cm) cucumber
- 2 avocados
- 3 $\frac{1}{2}$ ounces (100 g) baby spinach
- 10-13 fluid ounces (300-400 ml) water
- 2 tablespoons parsley, chopped
- $\frac{1}{2}$ bunch fresh basil
- 2 tablespoons chives, chopped
- $\frac{1}{2}$ tablespoon lime juice a pinch of salt

Directions

a) Cut up cucumber and avocado in large chunks.
b) In a blender or food processor mix spinach and water, starting with 10 fluid ounces (300 ml) of water.
c) Add remaining ingredients and blend again. Add more water little by little to get the right consistency, and taste to see if it needs more lime or salt.

41. Energy soup

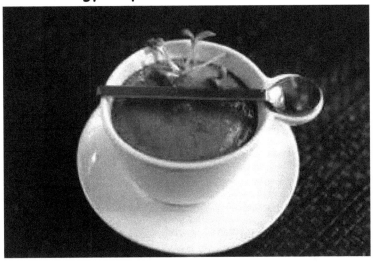

1 serving

Ingredients:

- 1 celery stalk
- 1 apple
- $\frac{1}{2}$ cucumber
- 1 $\frac{1}{2}$ ounce (40 g) spinach $\frac{1}{2}$ cup (100 ml) alfalfa sprouts tablespoons lemon juice
- $\frac{1}{2}$ -2 cups (300-500 ml) water
- $\frac{1}{2}$ avocado
- herbal salt to taste

Directions

a) Cut celery, apple, and cucumber into pieces.
b) Blend all ingredients except the avocado, starting with 1$\frac{1}{2}$ cup (300 ml) water. Add the avocado and blend again.
c) Add more water if needed and flavor with herbal salt.

SALADS

42. Cabbage with cranberry

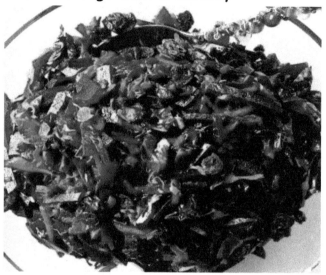

1 serving

Ingredients:

- ½ small head of cabbage
- 1 tablespoon olive oil
- 2 teaspoons lemon juice
- ½ tablespoon apple cider vinegar
- ½ cup (100 ml) cranberries, fresh or frozen and thawed
- ¼ cup (50 ml) pumpkin seeds, soaked

Directions

a) Shred the cabbage finely and place in a bowl. Pour in olive oil, lemon juice and apple cider vinegar.

b) Mix with your hands until the cabbage softens. Add the cranberries and pumpkin seeds and mix.

43. Spicy Vegetable Salad

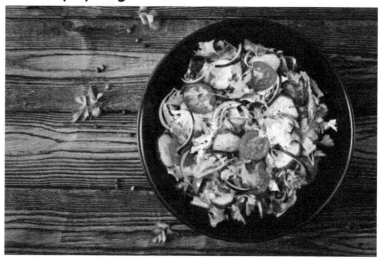

Ingredients

- spicy mix - heat oil, add mustard seeds, when they pop add cumin seeds then curry leaves and asafoetida
- Salt and sugar
- Lemon/lime juice
- Fresh coriander leaves
- Fresh grated coconut

Directions

a) Cut fresh vegetables and steam if needed.
b) Add any other ingredients to taste. Add the basic spicy mix at the end. (in a separate pan heat oil and add the spices, then add the mix to the vegetables)
c) Mix everything together and serve.

44.   Beetroot Salad

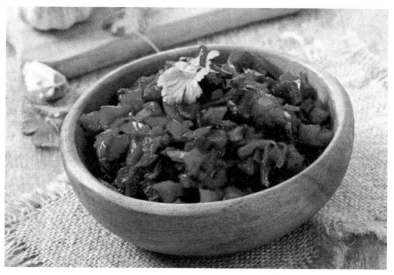

Ingredients

- 1/2 cup cooked beetroot – chopped
- 1 Tablespoon vegetable oil
- 1/4 Tablespoon mustard seeds
- 1/4 Tablespoon cumin seeds
- Pinch turmeric
- 2 pinch asafoetida
- 4-5 curry leaves
- Salt to taste
- Sugar to taste
- Fresh chopped coriander leaves

Directions

a) Heat oil then add mustard seeds.
b) When they pop add the cumin, then the turmeric, curry leaves and asafoetida.
c) Add spice mixture to beetroot along with the salt, sugar and coriander leaves to taste.

45.   Cabbage & Pomegranate Salad

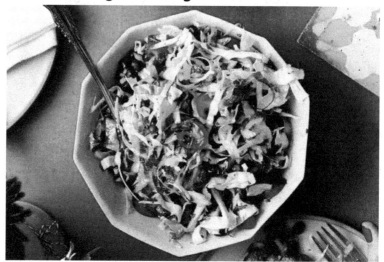

Ingredients

- 1 cup cabbage – grated
- $\frac{1}{2}$ pomegranate
- $\frac{1}{4}$ Tablespoon mustard seeds
- $\frac{1}{4}$ Tablespoon cumin seeds
- 4-5 curry leaves
- Pinch asafoetida
- 1 Tablespoon oil
- Salt and sugar to taste
- Lemon juice to taste
- Fresh coriander leaves

Directions

a) Remove seeds from the pomegranate.

b) Mix pomegranate with cabbage.

c) Heat oil in a pan and add the mustard seeds. When they pop add the cumin seeds, curry leaves and asafoetida. Add the spice mixture to the cabbage.

d) Add sugar, salt and lemon juice to taste. Mix well.

e) Garnish with coriander if desired.

46. Carrot & Pomegranate Salad

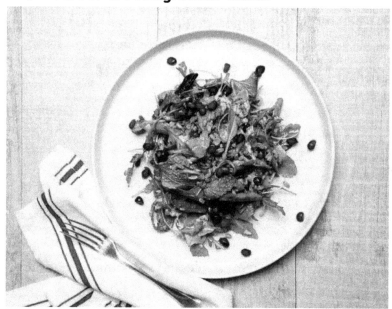

Ingredients

- 2 carrots – grated
- $\frac{1}{2}$ pomegranate
- $\frac{1}{4}$ Tablespoon mustard seeds
- $\frac{1}{4}$ Tablespoon cumin seeds
- 4-5 curry leaves
- Pinch asafoetida
- 1 Tablespoon oil
- Salt and sugar to taste
- Lemon juice – to taste
- Fresh coriander leaves

Directions

a) Remove seeds from the pomegranate.

b) Mix pomegranate with carrot.

c) Heat oil in a pan and add the mustard seeds. When they pop add the cumin seeds, curry leaves and asafoetida. Add the spice mixture to the carrot.

d) Add sugar, salt and lemon juice to taste. Mix well.

e) Garnish with coriander if desired.

47.   Cucumber Salad

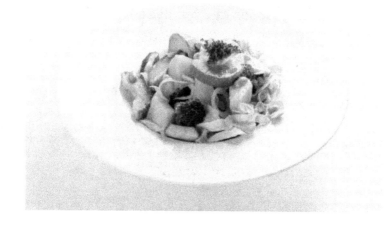

Ingredients

- 2 cucumbers – peeled and chopped
- Sugar and salt to taste
- 2 -3 Tablespoon roasted almond powder – or to taste
- 1 Tablespoon oil
- 1/8 Tablespoon mustard seeds
- 1/8 Tablespoon cumin seeds
- Pinch asafoetida
- 4-5 curry leaves
- Lemon juice – to taste

Directions

a) Heat the oil in a pan. Add the mustard seeds. When they pop add the cumin seeds, asafoetida and curry leaves.

b) Add the spice mixture to the cucumbers.

c) Add salt, sugar and lemon to taste.

d) Add the almond powder and mix well.

48. Hangover Helper Salad

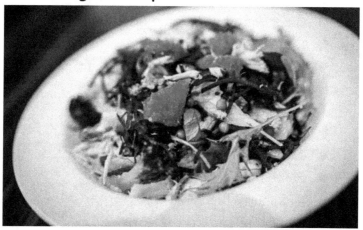

Ingredients:

- 3 cups chopped greens
- $\frac{1}{4}$ bulb of fennel, sliced thin
- $\frac{1}{2}$ cup chopped cooked broccoli florets
- $\frac{1}{2}$ cup chopped beets
- 1 to 2 tablespoons extra virgin olive oil
- Juice of $\frac{1}{2}$ lemon

Directions

a) In a large bowl, mix the greens, fennel, broccoli, and beets.

b) Toss with olive oil and lemon juice.

49. Pasta Toss

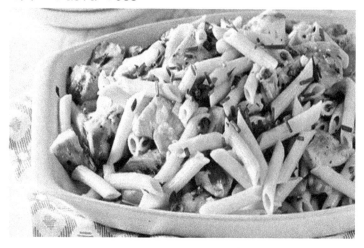

Ingredients:

- 1 (16-ounce) package pasta of your choice
- 1 tablespoon extra-virgin olive oil
- 2 cloves garlic, minced
- 1 (14-ounce) can artichoke hearts, drained and chopped
- Freshly ground black pepper, to taste

Directions

a) Bring a large pot of water to boil. Add pasta and cook according to package directions.
b) While pasta is cooking, heat oil in a large skillet over medium heat. Add garlic and heat for 1 minute. Add artichokes and cook until soft, about 7 minutes.
c) When pasta is cooked, drain and add directly to skillet. Toss with vegetables and season with black pepper, if desired.

50. Happiness Salad

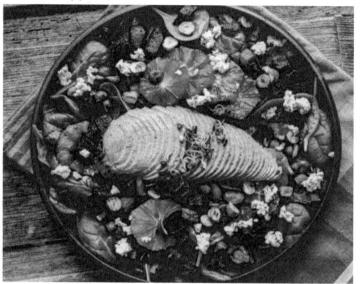

Ingredients:

- 2 cups baby spinach
- $\frac{1}{2}$ avocado, diced
- 1 cup beets, diced
- $\frac{1}{4}$ cup hazelnuts
- 2 tablespoons extra virgin olive oil
- 1 tablespoon balsamic vinegar

Directions

a) Put spinach, avocado, beets, and hazelnuts in a bowl. Dress with oil and vinegar.
b) Toss and enjoy.

51.   Daikon Radish Salad

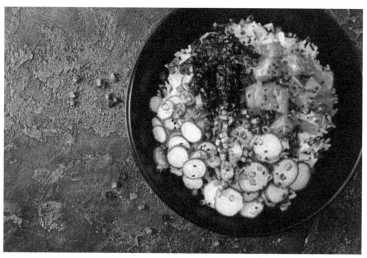

Ingredients
- 2 radish
- 3 Tablespoon roasted chana dal
- Lemon to taste
- 1/2 Tablespoon cumin seed powder
- Sugar to taste
- Fresh coriander leaves
- Salt to taste

Directions
a) Grate radish finely, including the green tops.
b) Add all ingredients and mix well.
c) Garnish with coriander.

52. Raw Pumpkin Salad

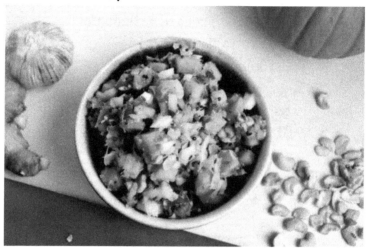

Ingredients

- 1 cup grated pumpkin
- $\frac{1}{4}$ Tablespoon mustard seeds
- $\frac{1}{4}$ Tablespoon cumin seeds
- 4-5 curry leaves
- Pinch asafoetida
- 1 Tablespoon oil
- Salt and sugar to taste
- Fresh coriander leaves

Directions

a) Heat oil in a pan and add the mustard seeds. When they pop add the cumin seeds, curry leaves and asafoetida.

b) Add spice mixture to the grated pumpkin.

c) Add sugar, salt to taste.

MAIN COURSE

53. Hangover shrimp

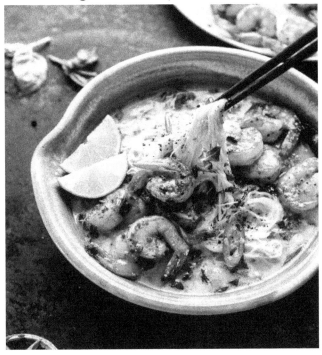

Yield: 1 Servings

Ingredient

- 32 ounces V-8 juice
- 1 can Beer
- 3 Jalapeño peppers (or habaneros)
- 1 large Onion; chopped
- 1 teaspoon Salt
- 2 Cloves garlic; chopped
- 3 pounds Shrimp; peeled and deveined

Directions

a) Place all ingredients, except shrimp, in a large pot and bring to a boil.
b) Add shrimp and remove from heat. Let stand about 20 minutes. Drain and chill shrimp.
c) Formatted and Busted by Carriej999@...

54. Lamb sausage rolls with harissa yogurt

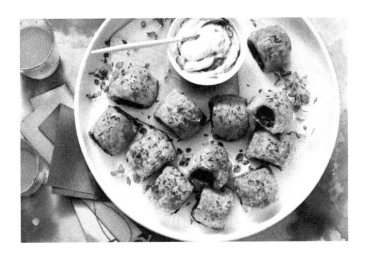

Ingredients

- 2 Tablespoons extra virgin olive oil
- 1 white onion, finely chopped
- 3 garlic cloves, crushed
- 1 Tablespoons finely chopped rosemary
- 1 teaspoon cumin seeds, crushed, plus extra
- 500g lamb mince
- 3 sheets frozen butter puff pastry, thawed
- 1 egg, lightly beaten
- 250g thick Greek-style yoghurt
- 1/4 cup (75g) harissa or tomato chutney
- Micro mint to serve (optional)

Directions

a) Preheat oven to 200C. Heat oil in a fry-pan over medium heat. Add onion and cook for 3-4 minutes until softened. Add the garlic, rosemary and cumin and cook 1-2 minutes until fragrant. Remove from the heat, chill for 10 minutes, then combine with mince.

b) Divide the mixture between pastry sheets, laying it along one edge to form a log. Roll to enclose, brushing the last 3cm of pastry overlap with egg-wash. Seal and trim pastry.

c) Place on a baking tray lined with baking paper, seam side down and freeze for 10 minutes. This will make them easier to slice.

d) Cut each roll into 4 and leave on the tray. Brush with egg-wash and scatter with extra cumin seeds. Bake for 30 minutes or until pastry is golden and rolls cooked through.

e) Swirl harissa through the yoghurt and serve with the sausage rolls, scattered with mint.

55. Madras butter chicken burger

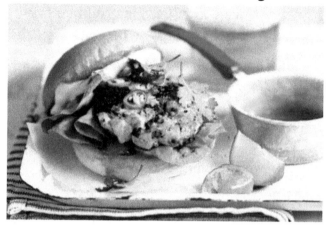

MAKES 6 BURGERS

Ingredients

- 2 (about 500g) chicken breasts, cut into 1cm cubes
- 1 Tablespoons hot Madras curry powder
- 1 Tablespoons nigella seeds
- 60g unsalted butter, chopped, softened
- 6 small white burger buns or bread rolls
- 2 Tablespoons mango chutney, plus extra to serve
- 1/2 cup (140g) Greek yoghurt
- 1/2 head butter lettuce, leaves separated
- Coriander leaves, to serve
- Thinly sliced long green chili (optional), to serve
- Lime wedges, to serve

Directions

a) Line a tray with baking paper and arrange egg rings on prepared tray. Place chicken, curry powder, nigella seeds and butter in a bowl and stir until chicken is well coated. Divide chicken mixture evenly among egg rings and chill for 2 hours or until patties are set.

b) Heat a non-stick fry-pan over medium-high heat. Add patties in their egg rings and cook for 4 minutes or until golden.

c) Flip patties and rings, and cook for a further 4 minutes or until patties are cooked through. Remove from rings and set aside, loosely covered with foil.

d) Split buns and spread chutney over bases and yoghurt over lids. Top each base with lettuce and a chicken patty. Sprinkle with coriander and chili, if using, and season.

e) Top burgers with bun lids and serve with extra mango chutney and lime wedges.

56. Quick chicken parmigiana

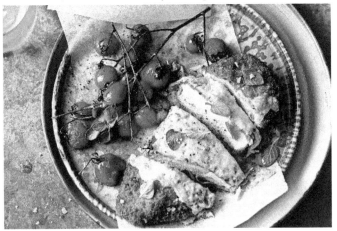

SERVES 4

INGREDIENTS

- 2 cups panko breadcrumbs
- 1 Tablespoons finely chopped thyme leaves
- 2 Tablespoons chopped oregano leaves, plus extra leaves to serve
- 1/2 cup (75g) plain flour
- 2 eggs, lightly beaten
- 4 x 180g chicken breasts
- Sunflower oil, to shallow fry
- 80g provolone cheese
- 500g vine cherry tomatoes
- Extra virgin olive oil to drizzle

Directions

a) Combine the panko, thyme, oregano and 1 teaspoon salt in a bowl then place the our and egg in separate bowls.

b) Flatten the chicken breasts slightly with a rolling pin, then individually coat in the flour, then the egg and then the panko mix.

c) Preheat oven grill to high.

d) Heat 11/2cm oil in a fry-pan over medium-high heat. Add the chicken and cook for 4 minutes a side or until golden. Drain on paper towel.

e) Place the chicken on a baking tray lined with baking paper. Top with torn pieces of cheese then add tomatoes to the tray, drizzle with a little oil and season.

f) Place under the grill and cook for 4-5 minutes until golden and bubbling and tomatoes are starting to collapse. Serve scattered with extra oregano.

57. Ultimate cheeseburger

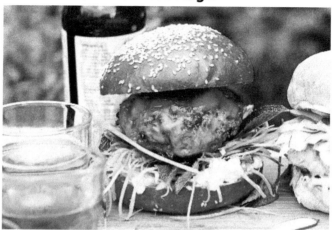

SERVES 4

Ingredients

- 700g coarsely ground chuck steak
- Extra virgin olive oil, to brush
- 4 slices tasty cheese
- 2/3 cup (190g) American mustard
- 4 milk buns, split, toasted
- 8 large dill pickles, sliced lengthways
- 2/3 cup (165ml) tomato sauce
- 1 small white onion

Directions

a) Season mince, then divide into four equal portions. Roll each into balls and flatten into four patties a little larger than buns (the meat will shrink during cooking). Chill for 30 minutes to firm up slightly.

b) Preheat a barbecue hotplate or large fry-pan to high heat and brush with oil. Season patties, then cook for 1-2 minutes on one side until well charred, then flip and place slices of cheese over each patty.

c) Cook for a further 1 minute or until cheese melts and patties are just cooked through. To assemble, spread half the mustard over the bun bases, then top with the patties, sliced pickles, tomato sauce and remaining mustard.

d) Sprinkle over onion, then top with bun lids to serve.

58. Moroccan lamb and harissa burgers

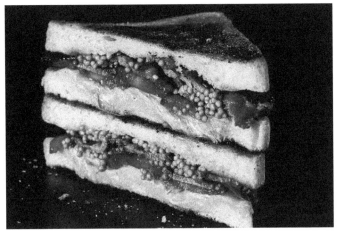

SERVES 4

Ingredients

- 500g lamb mince
- 2 Tablespoons harissa paste
- 1 Tablespoons cumin seeds
- 2 bunches heirloom carrots
- 1/2 bunch mint, leaves picked
- 1 Tablespoons red wine vinegar
- 80g red Leicester cheese, coarsely grated
- 4 seeded brioche buns, split
- 1/3 cup (65g) cottage cheese

Directions

a) Line a baking tray with baking paper. Place mince in a bowl and season generously. Add 1 Tablespoons harissa and, with clean hands, combine well.

b) Shape lamb mixture into 4 patties and sprinkle with cumin seeds. Place on prepared tray, cover and chill until needed (bring patties to room temperature before cooking).

c) Meanwhile, combine carrot, mint and vinegar in a bowl and set aside to pickle slightly.

d) Heat a barbecue or chargrill pan to medium-high heat. Grill patties for 4-5 minutes each side or until a good crust forms. Top with cheese, then cover (use foil if using a chargrill pan) and cook, without turning, for a further 3 minutes or until cheese has melted and patties are cooked through.

e) Grill brioche buns, cut-side down, for 30 seconds or until lightly toasted. Divide cottage cheese among bun bases, then top with pickled carrot mixture.

f) Add patties and remaining 1 Tablespoons harissa. Pop the lids on, squeezing so that the harissa oozes down the sides, and get stuck in.

59. Goat's cheese and maple bacon slice

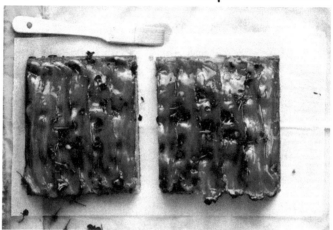

SERVES 6

Ingredients

- 2 2/3 cups (375g) white spelt flour, sifted
- 2 1/2 teaspoon lemon thyme leaves
- 1 1/2 teaspoon bicarbonate of soda, sifted
- 3 eggs, lightly beaten
- 3/4 cup (200g) thick Greek-style yoghurt
- 3/4 cup (185ml) extra virgin olive oil
- 150g goat's cheese, crumbled
- 300g streaky bacon
- 1/4 cup (60ml) maple syrup
- Micro purple basil, to serve

Directions

a) Preheat oven to 200°C. Grease and line a 20cm x 30cm slice pan with baking paper, leaving 5cm overhanging long sides of pan.

b) Combine flour, bicarb, 2 teaspoon lemon thyme and a pinch of salt in a bowl.

c) In a separate bowl, combine egg, yoghurt and oil. Using a fork, fold into dry ingredients and stir in cheese. Transfer to slice pan.

d) Trim bacon to 4cm longer than the width of the pan and arrange crossways on top, overlapping slices until slice is covered (bacon will shrink during cooking). Brush with 2 Tablespoons maple syrup, then bake for 30 minutes or until a skewer inserted into the centre comes out clean.

e) Preheat the oven grill to medium-high. Brush bacon with remaining maple syrup, scatter with remaining lemon thyme and grill for 90 seconds or until bacon is golden and bubbling.

f) Serve scattered with micro purple basil.

60. Asian-inspired fish burgers

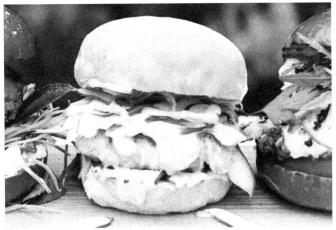

SERVES 4

Ingredients

- 500g skinless salmon fillets, pin-boned, cut into 1cm pieces

- 5cm piece (25g) ginger, finely grated

- 1 red chili, finely chopped

- 1/2 cup (25g) panko breadcrumbs

- 1 Tablespoons olive oil

- 4 soft white burger buns, split

- 1/2 Lebanese cucumber, peeled into ribbons

- 5 radishes, trimmed, thinly sliced

Chilli mayo

- 1/3 cup (100g) mayonnaise

- 1 Tablespoons chili sauce

Teriyaki mayo

- 1/3 cup (100g) mayonnaise

- 1 Tablespoons teriyaki sauce

Directions

a) Pulse half the salmon in a food processor until finely chopped. Add ginger and chili, and pulse briefly to combine. Transfer to a bowl, stir through remaining salmon pieces and season well with salt flakes and freshly ground black pepper.

b) Line a baking tray with baking paper. Divide salmon mixture into four 2cm-thick patties. Carefully coat the patties in breadcrumbs, pressing crumbs into the patties. Place on prepared tray, cover and chill for 20 minutes or until firm.

c) For the flavoured mayonnaise, combine ingredients for each mayonnaise in 2 separate bowls.

d) Heat a barbecue or chargrill pan to medium-high heat. Drizzle salmon patties with oil and cook, turning halfway, for 6-8 minutes or until golden and cooked through. Grill buns, cut-side down, for 30 seconds or until lightly toasted.

e) Place your burger bun bases on a serving platter. Divide cucumber among bases, top with salmon patties and radish, then spoon over the mayonnaise, letting them drizzle over the sides and onto the platter.

f) Top with bun lids and serve immediately.

61.   Korean Napa cabbage

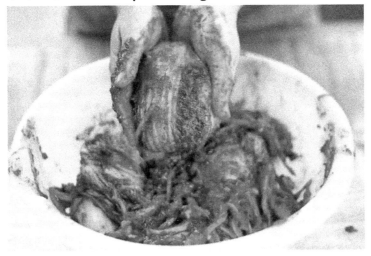

Ingredients

- outer leaves of napa cabbage, 300g

- Korean soybean paste, 5 Tablespoon

- garlic, 1 Tablespoon

- Korean soup soy sauce, 1 Tablespoon

- red chili powder, 1 Tablespoon

Directions

a) Put the outer leaves of a napa cabbage into boiling water and blanch it for 2 minutes with the lid open.

b) Rinse it in cold water. Gently squeeze the leaves to get rid of any remaining water.

c) Shred the cabbage into small pieces and put them into a large bowl. Add soy bean paste, garlic, soy sauce, red chili powder and mix well by hand.

d) Marinate for 10 minutes.

62. Korean Hangover Soup

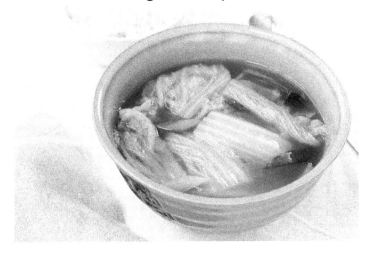

Ingredients

- beef bone broth, 1 litre

- beef flank or shank, diced 200g

- marinated napa cabbage

- sesame oil

Directions

a) Heat a deep pot over high heat. Add sesame oil and stir-fry the diced beef. Add napa cabbage and stir it with a large spoon for 20 seconds.

b) Add beef bone broth and boil for 20-30 minutes over medium high heat. Lower the heat and simmer for10 minutes.

c) Serve hot with steamed rice.

BEVERAGE

63. Caffeine-Less Yoga Tea

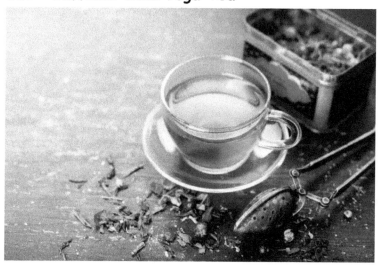

Ingredients:

- 10 ounces of water (about 1 1/3 cups)
- 3 whole cloves
- 4 whole green cardamom pods, cracked
- 4 whole black pepper
- $\frac{1}{2}$ stick cinnamon
- $\frac{1}{4}$ teaspoon chamomile tea
- $\frac{1}{2}$ cup almond milk
- 2 slices fresh ginger root

Directions:

a) Bring water to a boil and add spices.

b) Cover and boil 15 to 20 minutes, then add chamomile tea.

c) Let sit for a few minutes, then add the almond milk and return to a boil. Don't let it boil over.

d) When it reaches a boil, remove immediately from heat, strain, and sweeten with honey, if desired.

64. Artichoke Water

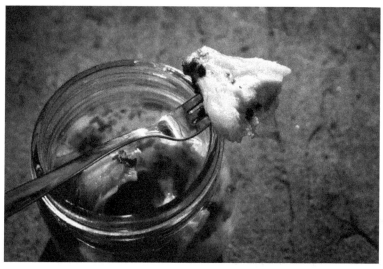

Ingredients:

- 2 artichokes

Directions

a) Cut the stems off the artichokes and cut the top inch off of the leaves.
b) Fill a large pot with water and bring to a boil. Add artichokes and boil for 30 minutes, or until you can easily pull off the bottom leaves of the artichoke.
c) Remove artichokes and save for a snack.
d) Let the water cool and then drink a cup of it.
e) This will help your liver detoxify itself and your entire body.

65. Virgin Mary

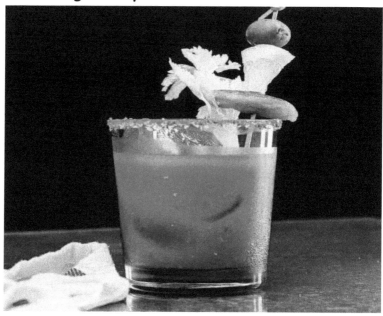

Ingredients

- 3 ounces tomato juice
- 1/2-ounce lemon juice
- 1 dash Worcestershire sauce
- 1 teaspoon celery salt
- Freshly ground black pepper
- 2 dashes hot sauce
- 1 stalk celery, for garnish
- 1 pickle spear, for garnish

Directions

a) Pour the tomato juice and lemon juice into a glass filled with ice cubes.
b) Mix well.
c) Add the Worcestershire sauce, salt, pepper, and hot sauce to taste.
d) Garnish with the celery stalk or pickle spear if using. Serve and enjoy!

66. Natural Vitamin Water

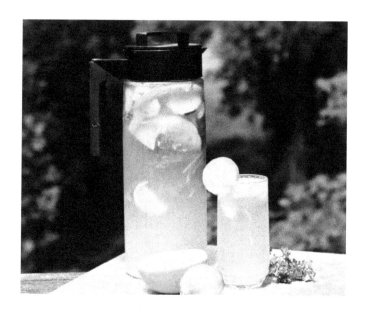

Serves 4

Ingredients
- Four cups of cold coconut or mineral water
- 1 lemon
- a handful of mint leaves
- slice of fresh ginger root
- 1 small cucumber
- handful of frozen raspberries
- handful of frozen blueberries
- optional: 1 Tablespoon of apple cider vinegar

Directions
a) Pour the water or coconut water into a jug and add the lemon, cucumber, mint leaves and berries.
b) Add a dash of apple cider vinegar if you're brave. Then let the water sit for about thirty minutes to allow the flavors to infuse into it.
c) Enjoy for a happy hangover!

67. Pineapple detox tonic in glass

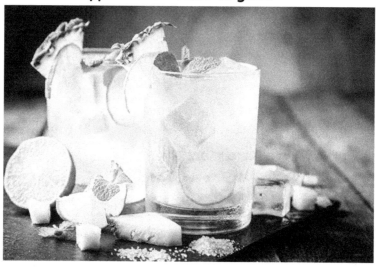

Ingredients

- 12 ounces raw coconut water
- 1/2 cup filtered water
- 1 green apple (cored and chopped)
- 1 cup fresh pineapple chunks
- Juice of 1 lime
- Juice of 1 lemon
- 1/4 cup fresh mint leaves
- 2 green apples (quartered)
- 3 cups fresh pineapple chunks
- 1 cup fresh mint leaves
- 1 lime (peeled and cut in half)
- 1 lemon (peeled and cut in half)
- 12 ounces raw coconut water
- 1/2 cup filtered water (optional)

Directions

a) Pour the coconut water and filtered water into the jar of a blender and add the remaining ingredients on top.

b) Blend on high speed until very smooth. The drink can be strained in a nut milk bag or sieve if you don't like pulp, but we love this drink as is fresh out of the blender.

c) This juice will hold for 24 hours in the refrigerator.

68. Ginger Tea

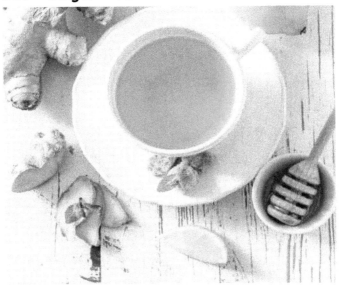

Yield: 1 cup

Ingredients

- 1-inch chunk of fresh ginger (no need to peel), sliced into pieces no wider than $\frac{1}{4}$-inch
- 1 cup water
- Optional flavorings (choose just one): 1 cinnamon stick, 1-inch piece of fresh turmeric (cut into thin slices, same as the ginger), or several sprigs of fresh mint
- Optional add-ins: 1 thin round of fresh lemon or orange, and/or 1 teaspoon honey or maple syrup, to taste

Directions

a) Combine the sliced ginger and water in a saucepan over high heat. If you're adding a cinnamon stick, fresh turmeric, or fresh mint, add it now.

b) Bring the mixture to a simmer, then reduce the heat as necessary to maintain a gentle simmer for 5 minutes (for extra-strong ginger flavor, simmer for up to 10 minutes).

c) Remove the pot from the heat. Carefully pour the mixture through a mesh sieve into a heat-safe liquid measuring cup, or directly into a mug.

d) If desired, serve with a lemon round and/or a drizzle of honey or maple syrup, to taste. Serve hot.

69. Blueberry & Spinach Smoothie

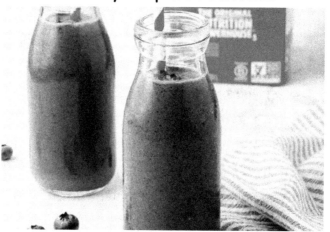

Servings 14

Ingredients

- 3 tablespoons old-fashioned oats
- 1 cup fresh spinach
- 1 cup frozen blueberries
- 1/3 cup plain Greek yogurt
- $\frac{3}{4}$ cup milk (whichever type you prefer)
- 1/8 teaspoon cinnamon (optional)

Directions

a) Place all ingredients in a blender and blend until smooth.
b) Serve immediately.

70. Pear Smoothie with Kale

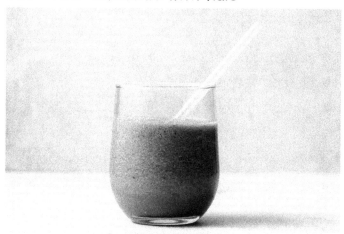

Yield: 4.75 cups

Ingredients

- ½ cup (120 ml) water
- 1 cup (150 g) green grapes
- 1 (130 g) medium oranges, peeled, quartered
- 1 (100 g) small banana, peeled
- ½ (90 g) Bartlett pear, cored
- 1 cup (60 g) kale
- 2 cups (260 g) ice cubes

Directions

a) Place all ingredients into the blender in the order listed and secure the lid.
b) Start the blender on its lowest speed, then quickly increase to its highest speed.
c) Blend for 45 seconds or until desired consistency is reached, using the tamper to press ingredients toward the blades.

71. Peanut Butter Protein Shake

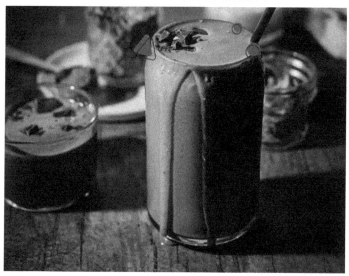

Ingredients

- 6 cubes ice cubes
- 1 cup milk
- 1 banana
- 1 scoop chocolate-flavored protein powder
- 2 tablespoons peanut butter
- 1 tablespoon honey
- 1 teaspoon unsweetened cocoa powder, or more to taste

Directions

a) Blend ice cubes, milk, banana, protein powder, peanut butter, honey, and cocoa powder together in a blender until smooth.

b) Enjoy.

72. Hangover Juice

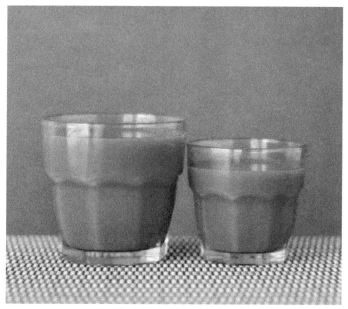

Ingredients

- 1 cup cauliflower
- 1 cup broccoli florets
- 1 apple, cored and quartered
- 1 orange, peeled

Directions

a) Blend the vegetables first, then the fruits.

b) Drink on your way to work, and you'll be feeling better within the hour! If your hangover persists, drink another glass.

73.   Berry Green

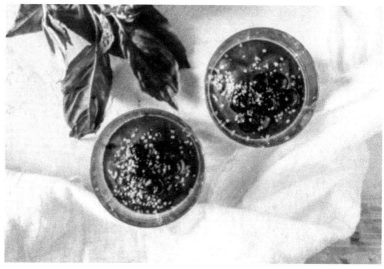

Ingredients:

- 3 handfuls spinach
- 2 cups water
- 1 apple, cored, quartered
- 1 cup frozen mango
- 1 cup frozen strawberries
- 1 handful frozen or fresh seedless grapes
- 1 stevia packet
- 2 tablespoons ground flaxseeds
- OPTIONAL: 1 scoop of protein powder

Directions

a) Place leafy greens and water into blender and blend until mixture is a green juice-like consistency.

b) Stop blender and add remaining ingredients. Blend.

74. Apple Strawberry

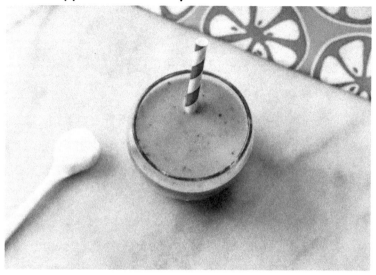

Ingredients:

- 3 handfuls spring mix greens
- 2 cups water
- 1 banana, peeled
- 2 apples, cored, quartered
- 1 $\frac{1}{2}$ cups frozen strawberries
- 2 stevia packets (add more to sweeten, if necessary)
- 2 tablespoons ground flaxseeds
- OPTIONAL: 1 scoop of protein powder

Directions

a) Place leafy greens and water into blender and blend until mixture is a green juice-like consistency.

b) Stop blender and add remaining ingredients. Blend.

75. Apple Berry

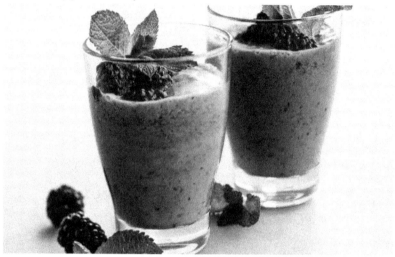

Ingredients:

- 1 handful spring mix greens
- 2 handfuls spinach
- 2 cups water
- 1½ cups frozen blueberries
- 1 banana, peeled
- 1 apple, cored and quartered
- 1 packet stevia
- 2 tablespoons ground flaxseeds
- OPTIONAL: 1 scoop of protein powder

Directions

a) Place leafy greens and water into blender and blend until mixture is a green juice-like consistency.

b) Stop blender and add remaining ingredients. Blend.

76. Berry Peachy

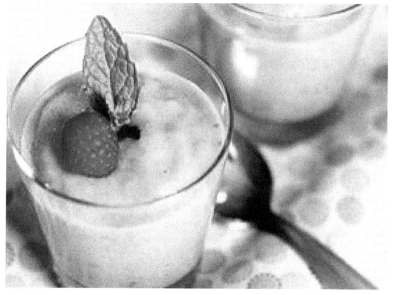

Ingredients:

- 2 handfuls kale
- 1 handful spinach
- 2 cups water
- 2 apples, cored, quartered
- 1½ cups frozen peaches
- 1½ cups frozen mixed berries
- 2 packets stevia
- 2 tablespoons ground flaxseeds
- 1 scoop of protein powder

Directions

a) Place leafy greens and water into blender and blend until mixture is a green juice-like consistency.
b) Stop blender and add remaining ingredients. Blend and Serve.

77. Peach Berry Spinach

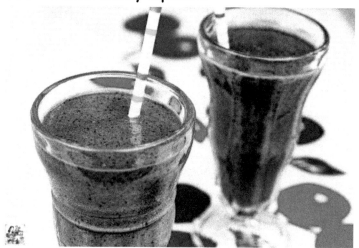

Ingredients:

- 3 handfuls spinach
- 2 cups water
- 1 cup frozen peaches
- 1 handful fresh or frozen seedless grapes 1½ cups blueberries
- 3 packets stevia to sweeten
- 2 tablespoons ground flaxseeds
- OPTIONAL: 1 scoop of protein powder

Directions

a) Place spinach and water into blender and blend until mixture is a green juice-like consistency.

b) Stop blender and add remaining ingredients. Blend and Serve.

78. Pineapple Spinach

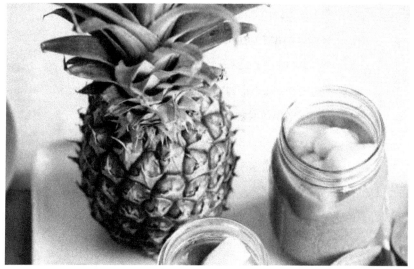

Ingredients:

- 2 cups fresh spinach, packed
- 1 cup pineapple chunks
- 2 cups frozen peaches
- 2 bananas, peeled
- $1\frac{1}{2}$ packets stevia
- 2 cups water
- 2 tablespoons ground flaxseeds
- OPTIONAL: 1 scoop of protein powder

Directions

a) Place spinach and water into blender and blend until mixture is a green juice-like consistency.

b) Stop blender and add remaining ingredients. Blend and Serve.

79. Pineapple Berry

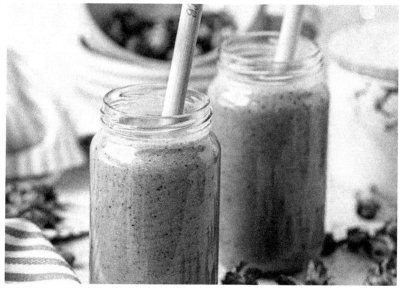

Ingredients:

- 2 handfuls spring mix greens
- 2 handfuls spinach
- 1 banana, peeled
- 1 $\frac{1}{2}$ cups pineapple chunks
- 1$\frac{1}{2}$ cups frozen mango chunks
- 1 cup frozen mixed berries
- 3 packets stevia
- 2 cups water
- 2 tablespoons ground flaxseeds
- OPTIONAL: 1 scoop of protein powder

Directions

a) Place leafy greens and water into blender and blend until mixture is a green juice-like consistency.

b) Stop blender and add remaining ingredients. Blend and Serve.

80. Lingonberry smoothie

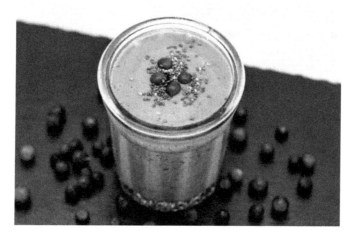

1 portion

Ingredients:

- 1-1½ cups (200-300 ml) water
- ½ cup (100 ml) almonds, soaked
- 2 apricots, soaked
- ¼ cup (50 ml) lingonberries, frozen or thawed

Directions

a) Blend together 1 scant cup (200 ml) water with almonds.

b) Strain through a mesh sieve.

c) Pour into the blender. Add apricots and blend again.

d) Blend in the berries and add more water to desired consistency.

81. Spinach Kale Berry

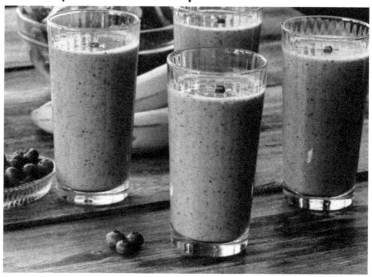

Ingredients:

- 2 handfuls kale
- 2 handfuls spinach
- 2 cups water
- 1 apple, cored, quartered
- 1 banana, peeled
- 1½ cups frozen blueberries
- 2 packets stevia
- 2 tablespoons ground flaxseeds
- OPTIONAL: 1 scoop of protein powder

Directions

a) Place leafy greens and water into blender and blend until mixture is a green juice-like consistency.

b) Stop blender and add remaining ingredients. Blend and Serve.

82. Apple Mango

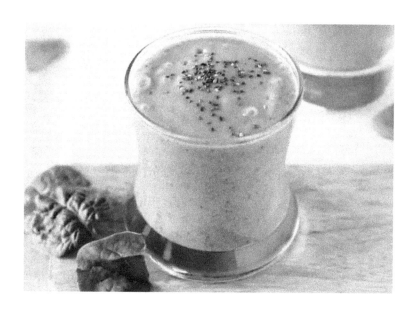

Ingredients:

- 3 handfuls spinach
- 2 cups water
- 1 apple, cored, quartered
- 1½ cups mangoes
- 2 cups frozen strawberries
- 1 packet stevia
- 2 tablespoons ground flaxseeds
- OPTIONAL: 1 scoop of protein powder

Directions

a) Place spinach and water into blender and blend until mixture is a green juice-like consistency.

b) Stop blender and add remaining ingredients to blender. Blend and Serve.

83. Pineapple Kale

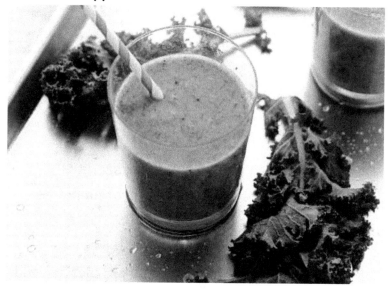

Ingredients:

- 2 handfuls kale
- 1 handful spring mix greens
- 2 cups water
- 1½ cups frozen peaches
- 2 handfuls pineapple chunks
- 2 packets stevia
- 2 tablespoons ground flaxseeds
- OPTIONAL: 1 scoop of protein powder

Directions

a) Place leafy greens and water into blender and blend until mixture is a green juice-like consistency.

b) Stop blender and add remaining ingredients. Blend and Serve.

84. Daily Lime & Dill Detox

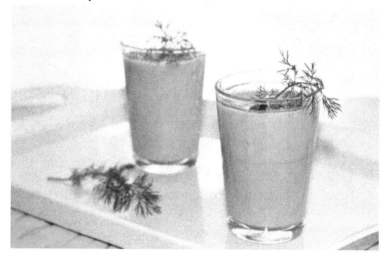

Serves: 2

Ingredients:

- 1/2 pear
- 1 cup chopped and seeded cucumber
- 1/4 cup chopped fresh dill
- 1 small avocado
- 1 cup baby spinach
- 2 tablespoons lime juice
- 1-inch knob fresh ginger-root, peeled
- 1 cup frozen pineapple
- 11/4 cups water
- 3 to 4 ice cubes

Directions

a) Place all the ingredients except the ice in a blender, and process until smooth. Add the ice and process again.
b) Drink chilled.

85. Peachy Kale Dream

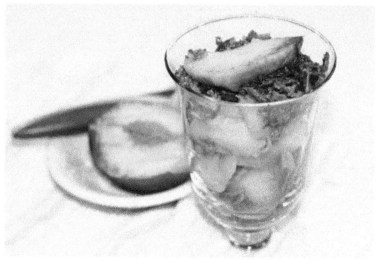

Serves: 2

Ingredients:

- 1/2 avocado
- 1 cup frozen organic frozen peaches
- 1 frozen banana, cut into pieces
- 2 tablespoons fresh lemon juice
- 11/4 cups water
- handful of kale
- 3 to 4 ice cubes
- Optional: 2 to 3 pitted dates

Directions

a) Place all the ingredients except the ice in a blender, and process until smooth.

b) Add the ice and dates (if using) and process again. Drink chilled.

86. Watermelon Cooler

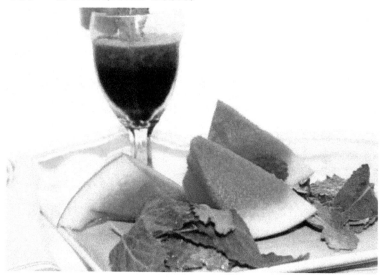

Serves: 2

Ingredients:

- 2 cups cubed seedless watermelon
- 1 whole cucumber, peeled, seeded, and coarsely chopped
- 1 large handful chopped kale
- 3 tablespoons fresh lime juice
- 1/4 cup chopped fresh mint
- 1/4 cup chopped fresh basil
- 1 cup ice cubes

Directions

a) Place the watermelon and cucumber in blender, and process until smooth.

b) Add the remaining ingredients and process again. Drink ice cold.

87.   Cinnamon Apple Smoothie

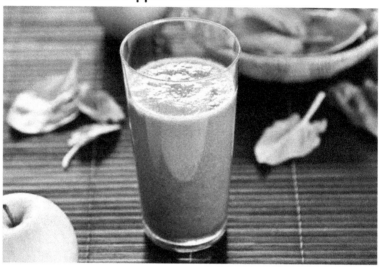

Serves: 1

Ingredients:

- 1 frozen banana, cut into bite-sized pieces
- 1 organic Granny Smith apple, cored and chopped (keep the skin on)
- 1 tablespoon fresh lemon juice
- 1 large handful baby spinach
- 1 cup cold water
- 2 to 3 pitted dates
- 1/2 teaspoon cinnamon
- 1/8 teaspoon nutmeg
- 4 to 5 ice cubes

Directions

a) Place all the ingredients except the ice in a blender, and process until smooth.
b) Add the ice and process again. Drink chilled.

88. Greeno-Colada

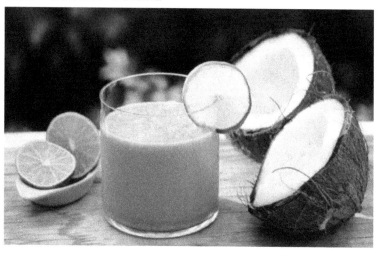

Serves: 1

Ingredients:

- 1 cup frozen chopped pineapple
- 3 tablespoons raw, unsweetened, shredded coconut
- 1 tablespoon fresh lime juice
- 1 handful baby spinach leaves
- 3 pitted dates
- 1 cup water
- 4 to 5 ice cubes

Directions

a) Place all the ingredients except the ice in a Blender, and process until smooth. Add the ice and process again.
b) Drink ice cold.

89. Mint Carob Smoothie

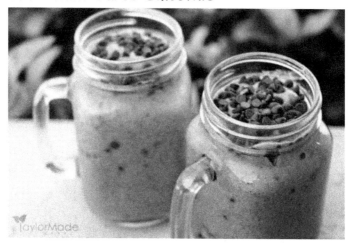

Serves: 2

Ingredients:

- 1 frozen banana, cut into bite-sized pieces
- 1/2 cup frozen peaches
- 1/2 cup raw macadamia nuts
- 1/3 cup chopped fresh mint leaves
- 3 tablespoons carob chips
- 2 to 3 pitted dates
- 1/2 teaspoon pure vanilla extract
- 11/2 cups water
- 3 or 4 ice cubes

Directions

a) Place all the ingredients except the ice in a Blender, and process until smooth.
b) Add the ice and process again. Drink chilled.

90. Sunny Delight Smoothie

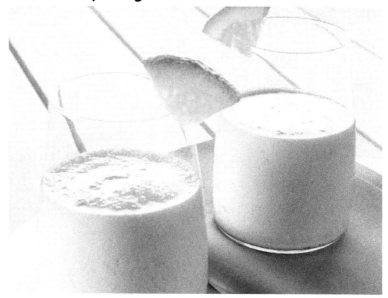

Serves: 1

Ingredients:

- 1 orange, peeled and chopped
- 1 kiwi, peeled and chopped
- 5 pitted dates
- 1/2 cup frozen pineapple
- 2 tablespoons hemp seeds
- 1/2 cup water
- 3 to 4 ice cubes

Directions

a) Place all the ingredients except the ice in a Blender, and process until smooth.

b) Add the ice and process again. Drink chilled.

91. Lime Smoothie

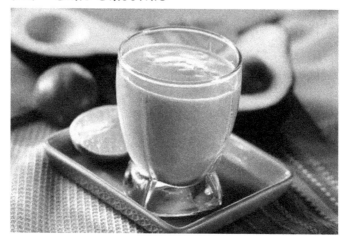

Serves: 2

Ingredients:

- 1 frozen banana, cut into bite-sized pieces
- 1/4 cup mashed avocado
- 2 tablespoons Nellie & Joe's Famous Key West Lime Juice
- 5 to 6 pitted dates
- 1/4 cup raw cashews
- 1/8 teaspoon pure vanilla extract
- 1/8 teaspoon unrefined sea salt
- 1 cup water
- 8 ice cubes

Directions

a) Place all the ingredients except the ice in a Blender, and process until smooth.
b) Add the ice and process again. Drink chilled.

92. Ginger & Wild Blueberry

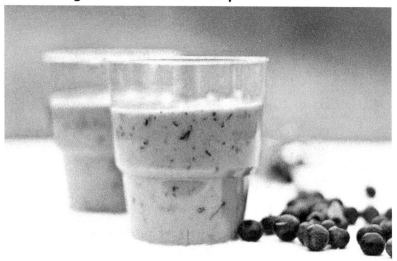

Serves: 2

Ingredients:

- 1 cup frozen wild blueberries
- 1/4 cup raw cashews
- 1 banana, cut into bite-sized pieces
- 1 tablespoon fresh lemon juice
- 1/2 teaspoon pure vanilla extract
- 1 tablespoon freshly grated ginger-root
- 5 to 6 pitted dates
- 1 cup cold water
- 5 to 6 ice cubes

Directions

a) Place all the ingredients except the ice in a Blender, and process until smooth.
b) Add the ice and process again. Drink chilled.

93. Cherry Vanilla Smoothie

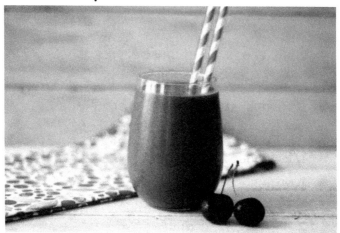

Serves: 2

Ingredients:

- 1 cup frozen pitted cherries
- 1/4 cup raw macadamia nuts
- 1/2 banana, cut into chunks
- 1/4 cup dried goji berries
- 1 teaspoon pure vanilla extract
- 1 cup water
- 6 to 8 ice cubes

Directions

a) Place all the ingredients except the ice in a Blender, and process until smooth. Add the ice and process again.

b) Drink ice cold.

94. Goji & Chia Strawberry bowl

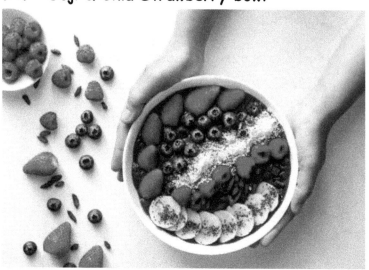

Yield: 1

Ingredients

- 1T goji berries
- 1T Strawberries
- 1-inch piece cinnamon stick
- 2-4T chia seeds
- 1 T coconut oil
- 16 oz. coconut water
- 1/3 c hemp seeds
- 2-3 large kale leaves
- 1c frozen berries
- ½ frozen banana

Directions

a) Place goji berries, cinnamon, and chia seeds in your blender, and add enough coconut water to cover well. Let soak about 10 minutes.

b) Add the remaining coconut water and the rest of the ingredients to the blender and process on the appropriate setting for smoothies, adding extra liquid for your desired consistency.

95. Slumbery Smoothie

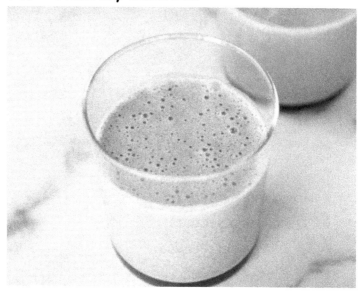

Ingredients:

- 2 cups baby spinach
- 1 cup almond milk
- 1 banana, peeled and sliced
- 1 teaspoon honey

Directions

a) Place all ingredients in a blender and puree.
b) Enjoy.

96.   Success Smoothie

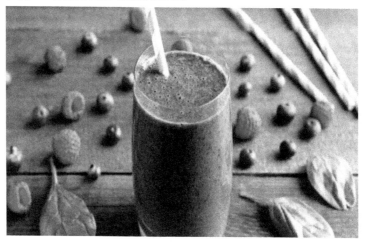

Ingredients:

- 1 cup strawberries, sliced
- 1 cup blueberries
- ⅓ banana, sliced
- 1 teaspoon ground flaxseeds
- 1 handful spinach
- 1 teaspoon honey

Directions

a) Blend everything together and enjoy!

97.   Green smoothie with figs

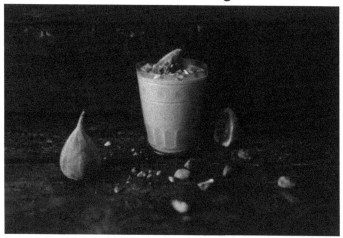

1 serving

Ingredients:

- 2.5 ounces (70 g) baby spinach
- 1½-2 cups (300-500 ml) water
- 1 pear
- 2 figs, soaked

Directions

a) Blend spinach with 1½ cups (300 ml) water.
b) Cut the pear, add along with the figs, and blend again.
c) Add more water if needed to find the right consistency for your smoothie.

98. Kiwi breakfast

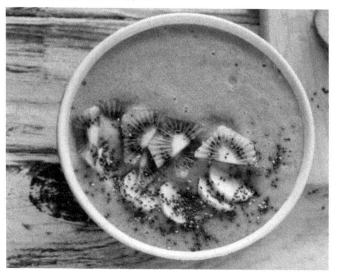

1 serving

Ingredients:

- 1 pear
- 2 celery stalks
- yellow kiwi fruits
- 1 tablespoon water
- $\frac{1}{2}$ teaspoon ground ginger

Directions

a) Cut pears, celery, and one of the kiwis into large pieces and mix in the blender with 1 tablespoon water until it is a smooth consistency.

b) Top with the other kiwi, cut into pieces, and ground ginger.

99. Zucchini, Pear & Apple Bowl

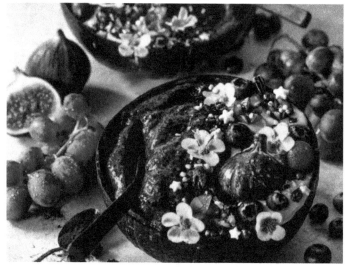

1 serving

Ingredients:

- ½ zucchini
- 1 pear
- 1 apple
- optional: cinnamon and ground ginger

Directions

a) Cut zucchini and pears into large chunks and blend in the food processor.
b) Add the apple, cut into large chunks, and continue blending to a smooth consistency.
c) Serve in a bowl and sprinkle with cinnamon and ginger.

100. Avocado and berries

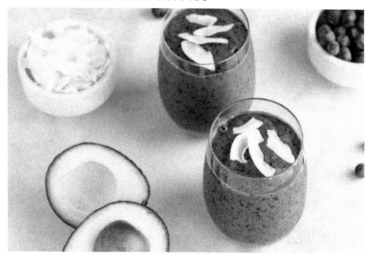

Ingredients:

- 1 avocado
- 1 pear
- 3½ ounces (100 g) blueberries

Directions

a) Cut the avocados and pears into pieces.
b) Mix together in a bowl and top with blueberries.

CONCLUSION

We all love a party, and that's fine but if you're having to pummel a hangover, it might be time to slow down the drinking, or even stop. But in any case, these recipes will be here for you, to cure that hangover!

CPSIA information can be obtained
at www.ICGtesting.com
Printed in the USA
LVHW081606300322
714783LV00002B/148